Prakriti

Your Ayurvedic Constitution

by

Dr. Robert E. Svoboda

Sadhana Publications
1998

This is a reference work.
It is not meant for diagnosis or treatment
and it is not a substitute for consultation
with a duly-licensed health care professional.

First published in the United States of America by
Geocom Limited

New ISBN 0-9656208-3-2
(Old ISBN 0-945669-00-3)

First Edition March 1988

Second edition November 1998

Sadhana Publications
1840 Iron Street, Suite C
Bellingham WA 98225

Dedication

This book is dedicated to my parents, who were my first teachers, and to Vimalananda, who was my friend, philosopher and guide.

It is also dedicated to Mother Tara, the Universal Mother Nature from whom we all originate, in whom we all exist, and to whom we all eventually return. She is the Mother of compassion, forgiveness, truth, beauty, knowledge, abundance, energy and freedom; She is equally well the Mother of darkness and bondage. From Her are born both sickness and health.

Motherliness is essential to healing because Mother Nature alone can heal. This book is humbly offered to Mother Tara with the request that She heal all of us, and heal our world.

Foreword

Ayurveda encompasses not only science but religion and philosophy as well. We use the word religion to denote beliefs and disciplines conducive to states of being in which the doors of perception open to all aspects of life. In Ayurveda the whole of life's journey is considered to be sacred. The word philosophy refers to love of truth, and in Ayurveda, Truth is Being, Pure Existence, the source of all life. Ayurveda, is a science of Truth as it is expressed in life.

Ayurveda believes that every individual is a unique phenomenon and that the individual is indivisible from the cosmos. Whatever is there in the macrocosm, the same thing exists in the microcosm. Every individual is a manifestation of cosmic consciousness.

The vibration of pure universal consciousness produces the soundless sound "Om." From this sound the five basic elements are produced: Ether, Air, Fire, Water and Earth. Furthermore, these five basic elements are manifested into the three biological organizations known as Vata, Pitta and Kapha. In every organism these three govern all physio-pathological changes.

At the time of fertilization, Vata, Pitta and Kapha determine by their permutations and combinations the constitution of an individual, which is called "- prakriti." The "prakriti" means "the first creation." Every human being is the first creation of the cosmos, and that is why every human being is a separate entity, a unique phenomenon. To understand this uniqueness of every individual is the study of "prakriti;" Ayurveda gives us a direct approach to this study.

The healing science of Ayurveda is based totally upon the knowledge of "prakriti," the individual constitution. If every individual knows his own constitution, then one can understand, for instance, what is a good diet and style of life for oneself. One man's food is another man's poison. Therefore, to make one's life healthy, happy and balanced, the knowledge of constitution is absolutely necessary.

My friend and colleague Dr. Robert Svoboda studied Ayurveda at the Tilak Ayurveda Medical College in Poona, India. There, he was a student of mine whose understanding and brilliance in Ayurveda resulted in his standing first in his class. This achievement is more noteworthy because Dr. Svoboda is an American who is the only Westerner to have ever completed the program in an Ayurvedic Medical School. His profound knowledge of Ayurveda and his background in English combine to make this important work of his invaluable to the Western reader.

Dr. Vasant Lad, October 1987

Author's Note

In the decade since this book first appeared many readers have sought me out to express their appreciation for its message. Gratifying as this praise has been, I have had to to temper it with a growing awareness that improvements to the book should be made. Hence this new edition, in which I have tried, by rewriting most of the original text, and adding new material throughout, to provide such improvements. New artwork honors Mother Nature perhaps more gloriously than before, and new editing has removed many older grammatical styles. I hope all readers will be pleased with the effort.

Acknowledgements

The author would like to thank the following people who read and critiqued this book, or otherwise offered assistance for its generation:

First Edition

Judy Allyn	Launette Rieb
Tyagi Kersten	Pamela Barinoff
Graham Dodd	Dr. Michael Stone
Elliot McLaughlin	Dr. Vasant D. Lad
Vaidya B. P. Nanal	Michael Laurenson
Fred & Kathy Smith	Dr. Greg Heil (Krsna Das)
Laura & Edwin Svoboda	Loretta Levitz & David Liberty
Vimalananda	Claudia Welch

Second Edition
Original artwork - Rhonda Rose
Editing - John Clancy
Page Layout - Ron Kozlowski

Table of Contents

Introduction

Nature and Her ways are truly inscrutable to mortals. You can set out on your life's journey intent on heading west, but if She wills you to go east your road will wind around until you are pointing eastward. When I left the U.S.A. on the Ides of March of 1973, I never suspected that I would end up living in India. What I expected was a brief African sojourn before returning to begin the September term at the University of Oklahoma Medical School.

A month later I was lying on my back in Abidjan, Ivory Coast, violently ill with dysentery. Two Frenchmen had taken pity on me and had brought me back to their apartment to spend the weekend until I could locate a doctor. They were themselves on their way to what they described as a "witch doctors' convention," a gathering of healers, magicians and trance mediums in the deep bush. Their guide was himself a "witch doctor." When he arrived and saw me lying inert on the bed utterly exhausted he insisted on treating me, and I was too weak to object.

He was a well-dressed young African of thirty-odd years with a robust physique who could easily have been mistaken for a bank clerk. Had I had the energy to think, I would have thought that he was a most unusual witch doctor. But I was too weak to think, and I thought nothing of it when he poured a glass of purified water from the carafe near my head and began to stare intently into it. I watched passively as he mumbled some sort of incantation over the glass and handed it to me to drink. I drank passively, assuring myself that mere water could do me no harm even if it did me no good. The doctor and the Frenchmen bade me adieu, and I sank into a profound sleep.

When I woke some hours later expecting to feel the dispiriting urgency of the disease I was pleasantly surprised to discover my abdomen calm. It remained calm all that day and the next, and would have continued to remain calm had I known then what I know now about the effect of diet on disease. But the lesson was well taken. A shaman had temporarily cured me, and with very little effort of faith on my part.

During my next few days of convalescence in that flat I also read *Autobiography of a Yogi,* which swung my internal compass around toward India. But first my steps led me to Kenya. There I participated with a team from the National Museum of Kenya on an ethnological expedition into the lands of the Pokot tribe. I was invited to join the tribe ritually, and did so. Once a Pokot, I interviewed tribal medicine men and women, and exchanged notes with our accompanying European M.D.s who testified to the usefulness of some of the tribe's traditional cures. Determined to study Pokot medicine more thoroughly, I promised myself to return to Kenya after a visit to South Asia.

I so hated India on first glance that I sprinted onward to Nepal, where the Peace Corps physician introduced me to the word Ayurveda. I returned to India in January 1974 only to attend a Tibetan Kalachakra initiation in Bodh Gaya at which the Dalai Lama officiated. The Kalachakra introduced me to the practical benefits of Yoga, and convinced me that despite any misgivings about India the society I had to remain there to study its ancient physical, mental and spiritual healing arts.

The Art of Medicine

One of the first things I learned in India was that medicine is an art. Until then I had looked at life mechanistically. I had viewed humans as thinking machines and disease and health as engineering problems. Ayurveda taught me that therapy becomes healing only when there is a healer involved. You can paint pictures, craft pots or compose concerti all day long, but unless you breathe life into your creations they will remain cold and lifeless. Knowing how to bring a creation to life is what separates a real artist from a mere artisan. Medical artists, men and women who marry their art to their science, make good medicine.

But Ayurveda (literally, "the science of life," or "the knowledge of living," or "the art of longevity") encompasses far more than mere therapeutic art. Ayurveda addresses everything that makes life worth living, like cookery. A well-tempered Ayurvedic physician must be a good cook to prepare good medicine. Hand-made Ayurvedic remedies usually outclass machine-made medicine, in the same way that the touch of a master chef's hand can convert an ordinary soufflé into something extraordinary. Most great chefs know nothing of the thermodynamics of food preparation; what they know is how to make their food delight the human palate. As a master chef is an artist of cuisine, so an Ayurvedic physician must become an artist of prescription. A good Ayurvedic physician has the same feel for her therapies that an expert cook has for his recipes. This feel, which develops as a physician attunes to Nature, is what transmutes a clinician's technical proficiency into intuitive healing. Ayurveda is not unscientific; it has progressed beyond mechanistic science.

No doctor since the beginning of time has ever cured a patient and no doctor ever will, for Nature alone can cure. Nature performs the miracles; doctors need only teach their patients how to tap into Nature's wonder working. Doctors should use what they can learn of a patient's past illnesses and present conditions to intuit future possibilities for health and establish healing strategies. True physicians offer themselves unceasingly as channels through which Nature can work Her magic. This is why Ayurveda teaches that every physician is immutably obligated to exert maximum energy for cure to all patients at all times, even during diagnostic procedures.

Despite its continual attention to cure when cure is what is needed, Ayurveda always emphasizes prevention over cure. Ayurveda balances and rejuvenates living organisms, reducing their susceptibility and empowering their immunity to prevent new disease from developing. Ayurveda is more a way of life, a way of learning how to cooperate with Nature and live in harmony with Her, than it is a medical system. Health in Ayurveda means harmony, and there is really no limit to the degree of balance that a sincere harmony-seeker can achieve.

Some complain that Ayurveda works slowly, but slowness is often part of the remedy, especially today when many of us suffer from the disease of haste. Human physiology has not changed much in recorded human history. Our technology is more advanced, surely, but our bodies and minds are almost identical to those of our ancestors, who suffered from the same diseases and demonstrated the same admirable and despicable qualities that we do.

What is different is that in ancient days, when Ayurveda was being developed, humans were much less able to control their external environments than we can today. They had no choice but to cooperate with and rely on Nature. Lacking fancy instruments, they cultivated their intuitive diagnostic abilities. Living in close proximity to Nature, they found that Nature Herself would tell them the medicinal effects of plants, animals and minerals if only they would listen closely to Her words. These early researchers experimented on themselves, each generation handing down its observations to the next. This collected medical lore was codified much later, but still long ago, in the form of Ayurveda.

Ancient Ayurvedists used their minds as computer systems, so developing their powers of memorization that they became storehouses of copious medical fact. Then they used their refined powers of intuition to apply what they had learned to their therapeutic interventions. They transformed Ayurveda into a healing art, and determined that the proper goal for any medical system should be no less than the achievement of immortality.

Health, Individuality, and Immortality

All humans have at one time or another dreamed of becoming immortal. Even though we know that everything that is created is eventually destroyed, each of us secretly cherishes the hope that Death might in our one case make an exception. India's ancient *rishis* (Seers) studied this question and addressed it in their hymns, which they collected into the oldest compositions of the human race, the Vedas. The Vedas, which are the foundation of Indian culture, emphasize that a potential for immortality is every individual's birthright. One famous Vedic prayer states:

> *Lead me from darkness into light.*
> *Lead me from untruth into truth.*
> *Lead me from mortality into immortality.*

Every embodied individual is composed of a body, a mind and a spirit. India's rishis therefore organized the wisdom, which became the Science of Life, into three bodies of knowledge. Ayurveda deals mainly with the physical body, Yoga deals mainly with the spirit, and Tantra is mainly concerned with the mind. All three disciplines share the same philosophy; differing emphases cause their manifestations to differ. Ayurveda is most concerned with life's physical bases, and concentrates on inducing right relationship of body with mind and spirit. Yoga controls body and mind to enable them to harmonize with spirit. Tantra uses the mind to seek to balance the demands of body and spirit.

We all exist as individuals against the background of our external environment, Mother Nature. None of us can ever be wholly individual, for Nature conditions our individuality. Most of us embrace the world, indulging ourselves unlimitedly, relying on the world to continue supplying goodies to us and on Nature to provide us enough digestive power to consume them. Most of us call this self-indulgence freedom.

True freedom is, however, the ability to be totally adaptable. Enjoyment is certainly one of life's purposes, but you lose your ability to enjoy when you exceed your limits. Limitation is inherent in life. You are limited by dozens of obligations, such as the necessity to breathe, to eat, to sleep, and to use words to communicate with others. Your most important limitation is your organism's capacity to endure your indulgences.

Either you can willingly limit yourself or Nature will limit you. Disease is Nature's way of forcing you to slow down and rest. This is why She is called Mother Nature: She loves you so much that She cannot bear to see you ruining yourself. She warns you of your errors over and over, and turns to drastic measures only when you obstinately refuse to listen to Her. It is a classic case of freedom versus responsibility: either you restrict your freedom a little bit each day, or Nature will come along and restrict it for you for days, weeks or months at a time.

Indulgence is a legitimate life goal, but it is only one of four life goals. No life is completely lived unless each of these goals is achieved. They are:

>**Dharma,** the goal of fulfilling the duties assigned to us by our positions in society;
>
>**Artha,** the goal of accumulating possessions in the course of fulfilling our duties;
>
>**Kama,** the goal of satisfying legitimate desires with the assistance of one's accumulated possessions; and
>
>**Moksha,** the goal of realizing that there is more to life than duty, possessions and desires.

You need a stable niche in society in order to arrange for the necessities of life and the leisure to permit you to live either a life of indulgence or one of spiritual asceticism. Whatever your life aim you need a sound mind in a sound body to achieve it. You have to be healthy if you want to enjoy yourself continuously.

The rishis designed Ayurveda especially for those individuals who want to enjoy the world healthily. Ayurveda's daily and seasonal routines, dietary guidance, therapeutics and doctrine of antidotes for the side-effects of addictions can keep you hale, hearty and having a high time well into your senescence if you can restrict yourself sufficiently to follow these precepts strictly. You must consciously choose how much you wish to indulge, which will determine how healthy you will be. There is no free lunch.

Some people think they have found a free lunch in Tantra, which transmutes an individual's relationship to external inputs so that he or she can take or leave them at will. Though Tantra seems to provide unlimited indulgence under the cover of spirituality it is in fact an exceedingly rigorous system which can be successfully begun only after strenuous Ayurvedic purification and Yogic practices. Yoga traditionally encourages people to keep the world at arm's length, to live ascetically in order to limit the introduction of external disturbances into their internal environments. Yoga and Tantra help make an individual independent of dependence on the world, but their practices cannot be safely followed without at least a rudimentary knowledge of Ayurvedic principles and practices.

Individual balance or harmony has a vertical dimension that is the dynamic interplay of the individual's body, mind and spirit; its horizontal dimension is the equilibrium between the individual and his or her environment. Your physical body must be in balance with Nature, your mind must be in harmony with the group-mind of the society or group you live in, and your soul must be in a satisfying relationship with the Universal Soul if you are to be truly healthy. The rishis used all life as their textbook; physicians must do the same, learning for themselves when and how it is appropriate to deal with a patient's body, mind or spirit.

It is easiest to harmonize the body-mind-spirit complex by starting with the body, which is relatively stable. Balance of the mind and spirit, which are ethereal and therefore inherently difficult to stabilize, comes more easily once the body has been made firm and healthy. This is especially important today when most people are thoroughly enthralled with the material world. A physician must treat a patient at the level of consciousness on which the patient can respond, and since most people are submerged in physical consciousness, physical medicine should be first employed. Occasion to use mental and spiritual medicine inevitably follows.

Every human being is a unique individual, full of idiosyncrasies and peculiarities. Your most precious possession, your life, is yours and yours alone, unlike that of any other human being past, present or future. Each human is a unique manifestation of Mother Nature, the Creative Energy of the universe. Each possesses an indwelling fragment of the Universal Soul. The message of the Vedas is that each of us must find our own path to a life lived to the fullest, for only by making the most of ourselves can we repay to Nature the debt we owe Her for giving us life. The universe needs you to add your mite to the vast collective tapestry we call human civilization. You can make your fullest contribution to life only when you are healthy and health alone enables you to enjoy your life to the fullest in return.

The word Svastha means "healthy" in Sanskrit. Sva ("self") + Stha ("established) = Svastha ("established in the self"). The "self" here is the ego, not the Freudian ego but the power of individual identity, which separates every being from every other being. The ego is that which gives me my identity, which makes me me, which causes me to know that I am I and not you, he, she, we or they. This power which perpetually reminds me that I am I is called in Sanskrit *ahamkara* (literally, "the I-former"). Because each of us is a body, a mind and a spirit, we each have a body-I, a mind-I and a spirit-I. To be "established in self" is to be established in each of these selves.

Today's physicians tend to ignore individuality. They often look at people as "livers" or "lungs," and neglect the organism that hosts that liver or lung. Some espouse the therapy they know best as a cure-all for all the ailing, overlooking the variations which exist even among patients of the same illness. Such piece-meal therapy cannot encourage balance in the organism. Since today's doctors often fail to project health onto their patients, today's patients must learn to project health themselves. Everyone in today's world who wants to be healthy has a personal responsibility to learn as much as possible about health.

Many Westerners will study Ayurveda in hopes of finding miracles that will allow them to continue to go about their self-indulgent ways. Though they may find temporary relief this way, permanent relief will come only with permanent changes in lifestyle. These people cheat themselves in the same way that people who flock after miracle-mongers in hope of effortless spiritual advancement cheat themselves. Ayurveda is designed for those who are ready to take responsibility for themselves.

If Ayurveda were a religion Nature would be its Goddess, and overindulgence would be the sole sin She would punish. Ayurveda is meant to allow you to enjoy the pleasures of life up to the point that such enjoyment interferes with your health. Full-time gratification is in fact bondage, because the more we consume the more we become captives of our consumption. Unlimited indulgence makes us less free because we become less self-sufficient. Each of our addictions—to caffeine, sugar, salt, sports spectaculars, TV game shows, alcohol, drugs, gambling palaces or other indulgences—is another nail in the coffin of our freedom, another restraint to our individual freedom. Most of us don't even know how to indulge properly, and we sicken and die from the side effects of our indulgences. True enjoyment is possible only where there is true health.

As I have traveled around the world I have talked to people about Ayurveda, trying to discover what Ayurveda can do for them. This book is one result of my travels. It is not an exposition of the classical principles of Ayurveda; in fact, an old-line Ayurvedic physician might well take issue with me over some of the points that I make. It is instead my own interpretation of certain Ayurvedic theories. I am indebted to my teacher Vimalananda for these observations, for it was he who taught me to think in this way.

Darshana, the Sanskrit word for "philosophy," literally means "seeing." Philosophy is that which allows you to see things in a certain way. Ayurveda is a philosophy which allows physicians to see patients the way Nature sees them. The sages who created Ayurveda were called "Seers" because of their

6

ability to perceive reality clearly. They could see how the world and its parts operate, and described their observations in words which allowed those who came later to see and perceive in similar ways. Since each Seer saw things from a different viewpoint there are many systems of Ayurveda, not just one. Following this tradition every Ayurvedic physician has his or her individual system, derived from the experiences of the Great Seers and augmented by personal experience.

This book is a partial exposition of my own experience. It begins with an introduction to the fundamentals of the Ayurvedic worldview and shows how these principles determine constitutional types. It proceeds to consider the effects of food on constitution, the inner nature of nutrition, and good habits for establishing and preserving health.

The subject matter then strays into topics that explore the forces that bind body, mind and spirit together, concentrating on ahamkara and the nature of individual identity. You are healthy (svastha) when you are established in your self, and we examine how establishment in self comes about, how it is maintained, and how it is upset. The book introduces Ayurveda's explanation of disease causation, and presents examples of the Ayurvedic approach to disease management and rejuvenation, including some esoteric methods of self-balance.

Many Sanskrit tomes open with the word "atha," which means "now," indicating that the book's knowledge is waiting within ready to be experienced at any time by anyone who opens it. Ayurvedic knowledge is perennial and universal, as valid today as it was 5,000 years ago and as it will be 5,000 years from now. Details may change and specifics may come and go but the essence of the knowledge remains inviolate. Ayurveda's unbroken chain of expertise both in delivering therapies and in determining the appropriate therapy for each condition have been tested by thousands and thousands of physicians on millions and millions of patients. Its theories and practices have both stood the test of time.

I have studied Ayurved's ancient writers like Charaka, Sushruta and Vagbhata both in translation and in the original Sanskrit. Taking their teachings to heart I have tried to apply the essence of their ancient wisdom to the specifics of our modern problems. Ayurveda can be quite complex, and I have taken the liberty of extracting from it a few teachings which I feel can act as initial tools for those of us who want to improve ourselves.

One major modern problem is rootlessness, a disease that is promoted by the great mobility of today's people. We Americans pride ourselves on the fluidity of our culture, which is the world's melting pot. Ours is a society in which everyone can (theoretically) use talent and ambition to earn fame and fortune. Every man a king, at least of himself, is our motto. We revel in our rootlessness, and love to live footloose, free of all ties and limitations of the past. Most of our ancestors came from other countries to forget their pasts, and forgetting the past has become an American rite of passage. In magnifying our individuality thus we came to equate progress with forgetfulness, and now

Progress (as epitomized by Science) has become our idol. Most of us today live our lives as slaves to Progress.

Allegiance to progress makes us tend to confuse individuality with sovereignty. A strong sense of individual identity is important to the health of all humans, but in older societies in which all members shared a culture an individual was not solely responsible for defining his or her identity. The Japanese, for example, know that they have inherited the ancient culture of Japan. Much of their personalities depend on the extent to which they adopt or reject the tenets of that culture.

America's cultural institutions are much less deeply ingrained in us, and Americans are in general much less willing to respect the past than are other peoples. Since we have less past experience for soil in which to plant the seeds of our personalities we must rely more on our own individual experience. Each of us egoically establishes an individual ethic and morality. Unfortunately, most of us invest a lot in our individualities, since we have nothing else to invest in with confidence. We have a collective policy of *sauve qui peut* (everyone for oneself) which regards everything outside the individual, even Nature, as an enemy.

> Forgetfulness is a devastating disorder. We modern humans have forgotten our roots, we have forgotten our gods, and we are now busily trying to forget our morals. We feel freer and less constrained the more we forget, unaware that each additional loss of memory distances us further from our true identities. We construct for ourselves false personalities derived from the veneer of addictions to our sensory indulgences, defining freedom as unlimited gratification, forgetting that all individuality is conditional. Cut off from communication with our internal mother we are severed from our source of compassion, and we forget how to empathize with other living creatures.

This is why many of us do not hesitate to eliminate anything which is either not part of us or has no demonstrable benefit to us. Thus our society is violent. Our literature, our art, our music, even our agriculture is violent, and our medicine is equally violent. We kill with antibiotics and antiseptics, and if our slaughter is ineffectual we use surgery to expel the offending organ from our presence. We destroy the body in order to save it.

"Establishment in the self" cannot however mean cutting yourself off from your source, the being Who has created you. Overinvestment in self is as unhealthy as its opposite. Destruction should be a last resort; nurturance, a motherly feeling of nurture and support for oneself and for all beings, should be the first resort. Nature is always magnanimous, and She will be as generous to you as you are generous to yourself and to other beings. You cannot buy, beg, borrow or steal health; it is Nature's gift to you.

Ayurveda is the product of a civilization that is deeply rooted in Mother Nature. The Seers knew that all of Nature is part of the individual, since we all are created from, exist in, and return to Nature. Individuality is thus a very temporary condition that can flourish only with Nature's assistance, not Her enmity.

Carl Jung expressed this opinion after a visit to India in 1938:

"It is quite possible that India is the real world, and that the white man lives in a madhouse of abstractions.... Life in India has not yet withdrawn into the capsule of the head. It is still the whole body that lives. No wonder the European feels dreamlike; the complete life of India is something of which he merely dreams. When you walk with naked feet, how can you ever forget the earth?"

This book aims to reintroduce Westerners to "walking with naked feet" through life, that they may renew their contact with Nature. The concept of individual constitution is, though centuries old, a new concept for the Western mind, a new way for us to understand our relationship with Nature.

Ayurveda is above all meant for all people who by harmonizing themselves seek to act as harmonizing forces in the universe. Our overweening, arrogant passion for self-indulgence has poisoned our world. If we hope to continue to live on this planet we must reverse the damage that we have inflicted on ourselves and on our environment. We must calm Nature's ire if we want Her to return us to health. Vimalananda often said that the purpose of the Science of Life is to make every home a happy home, a home in the true sense of the word: a haven. Everyone should have a real home, a haven they can always go home to, inside and outside themselves. All of us have a Mother in Nature, and only She can lead us home.

Chapter One
Doshas and Tastes

Each of us maintains separateness from other living beings for as long as Nature permits us to remain alive. Nature gives us the space bounded by the skin and the digestive tract to call our own. Every thing outside your skin is part of your environment. You are a part of my environment, and I am a part of your environment. Nature is the sum total of all individuals and their environments.

Inside your digestive tract is material that was originally part of your environment. Where once it had its own separate existence, its own individuality, now it is on metabolic probation, attempting to pass the digestive exams to become a part of you. Until it passes those exams it remains alien to you. Should your gastrointestinal tract rupture some of this material will escape into your body cavity. Your body will recognize it as alien and react to it, a reaction that if allowed to progress will kill you very quickly.

When your external skin fail to do its job, as might occur after severe burns, alien marauders enter your system from without, which may also result in your demise. We owe our continued day-to-day existence to the admirable fortitude of our twin boundaries: the body's external skin and the internal skin of the gut.

Diseases are beings with parasitical intentions. Some have collective bodies, like worms, bacteria and viruses, and show the same signs of collective consciousness that social insects like ants and termites do. Other diseases which have no bodies of their own "take possession" of an organism in order to express the compulsions of their individual existences. Still others entities, like cancer, are created within the body. Whatever the intruder, cure occurs when the alien personality is expelled from the organism and the host's innate personality returns to normal.

Aliens are unwelcome in a healthy body. An unbalanced system invites them in by encouraging improper digestion of food. Poor digestion produces a variety of physical and mental toxins collectively called *ama* in Sanskrit. Ama acts as food for parasites, encouraging them to thrive in the organism. Indigestion develops through poor eating and living habits. This sort of deliberate, willful indulgence in unhealthy practices is called in Sanskrit *prajnaparadha* ("crimes against wisdom").

Indigestion prevents nutrients from reaching the tissues, and weakens the host's immune defenses. The human aura is our first line of defense against parasitical beings. The skin and the gut form the second line of defense. A third line of defense, the immune system, waits to intercept and destroy any parasites that somehow find their way past the first two defenses. The immune system, which communicates with both the skin and the gut, is a sense organ with a "sixth sense" for intruders. The immune system is an intricate web of T-cells, B-cells, antibodies and lymphokines, a system of fascinating complexity all controlled by a single boss: *ahamkara*.

Ahamkara ceaselessly identifies itself with each of the trillions of cells in the body. Your ahamkara constantly reminds every one of your cells of its identity as a sub-unit of that grand and glorious entity known as **You**. Ahamkara ensures that only those cells that swear allegiance to her lordship are allowed to remain alive in the body. All aliens are hunted down and ruthlessly slaughtered, and all rebels—mutant or cancerous cells—are mercilessly executed as a warning to other cells that might dare to resist her rule.

You can remain alive, safe inside your castle, only so long as your ahamkara serves as your garrison governor. When she is injured, alien beings may find a weak spot in your defenses and strike you down. When she, the warder who forces your cells to slave away for you, relinquishes her charge, all the inmates are free to go their own ways, and you die. She is your wife, your lover, your friend, your guide and advisor, your servant. She is your all-in-all. Above all, she is your mother.

Ahamkara is feminine because she is a fraction of the Divine Mother Goddess Nature. She is your wife because she is always with you, bonded in the marriage of body to mind to soul which is you. She is your lover because only the power of her love can bind all your cells together and induce them to function in concert as a unified being. She is your friend because she is always there to sympathize with you. She guides and advises you regarding your self-interest. As servant, she tirelessly slaves away to keep you running.

This "I-former" is your mother because she aggregates to herself all the building blocks that form you: the Five Great Elements, the sense organs and the mind. The ancient *rishis*, who knew this "I am" principle well, worshipped their own ahamkaras as mothers that they might enter into loving relationships with them. India is a motherland because the rishis recognized in their transcendent wisdom the creative importance of Mother Nature. Even Adi Shankaracharya, the originator of ten sects of renunciate monks who shun all normal human interactions, mandated worship of the Great Goddess in all his monasteries.

Diseases arise when ahamkara is afflicted and immunity weakens. The Sanskrit word for immunity is *vyadhikshamatva*, which literally means "forgiveness of disease." You retain your health only so long as you are willing to forgive your stresses, shrug off adversity and adapt to new situations. Resistance to change always impedes the workings of your immunity. An old Sanskrit proverb tells us *kshama cha janani*: the essence of motherly love is forgiveness. Damage to the ahamkara-mother predisposes us to disease by weakening our innate forgiveness.

Treatment of ahamkara is the ultimate medicine. India's sages have long known that good spiritual health is a prerequisite for good physical and mental health. Spiritual health is a dynamic balance between a strongly integrated individual personality and the cosmic personality of Nature, a balance that is possible only so long as a being remembers its debt to Mother Nature.

Only immortal beings can be completely healthy; only they have so empowered their own ahamkaras that no alien being can ever invade them. India's ancient rishis performed long penances to completely awaken and control their ahamkaras, and they became immortal in consequence. Their desire to communicate their experiences to others led them to establish the system of philosophical "seeing" which students of Ayurveda use to look at embodied life.

When the wise rishis examined their own experience and consulted their intuitions they realized that human consciousness, will and identity must be fragments of Nature's own consciousness, will and identity. The subtlety of their faculties of perception permitted them to contact Nature and communicate with Her directly. One of the first things they learned concerned the structure and origin of the universe.

Nature told them that first exists

Pure Existence,
The One Without a Second.

When within Pure Existence a desire for manifestation arises

Consciousness and Will appear.

These two mate together. Their offspring is

Intellect,

the power of discrimination.
Intellect then individualizes itself into

Ahamkara,

the "I-former." The universe fills with numberless little individual bundles of - intellect all searching for a means of expression. According to their innate predilections these ahamkara-bundles manifest as:

waves of kinetic energy known as *Rajas,*

material particles of potential energy known as *Tamas,*

and the subjective consciousness known as *Sattva*

Rajas is activity and Tamas inertia. Sattva is the balance of these two, for only consciousness can balance kinetic energy with potential energy. Nature's ahamkara is sufficiently vast to balance the energies of the entire cosmos. The power of the I-consciousness in humans is sufficient to balance their own individual energies.

An individual bundle of "spirit," desirous of expressing itself, uses subjective consciousness (Sattva) to manifest sense organs and a mind. Spirit and mind then project themselves into a physical body, created from the Five Great Elements that arise from Tamas. The sense organs use Rajas to project from the body into the external world to experience their objects. The body is the mind's vehicle, its instrument for sense gratification. The mind retreats to its bodily haven each night during sleep when it is tired of roaming about outside. The spirit remains within this haven at all times, providing life to the body and consciousness to the mind.

The Five Great Elements

Just as our bodies are made up of trillions of independent cells, we are all little cells in the universal organism. Like our cells, each of us humans has an individual existence but none of us is "free" enough to live independently of the whole. In fact, everything which exists in the external universe has its counterpart in a living being's own personal internal universe. Every cosmic force is represented, in altered form. The flow of nutrients into and wastes out of body cells also characterizes the continuous flow of nutrients and wastes into and out of plants, animals and humans.

There is therefore no inherent difference between, say, cooking your food in a pot on the stove and cooking your food in the pot of your stomach on the stove of your internal digestive "fire." Both use heat to prepare the food for easier assimilation. Flames are used on the external stove and acid and enzymes on the inside, but the principle of cooking is identical to both.

The rishis used the theory of the Five Great Elements (which are more properly known as the Five Great States of Material Existence) to explain how these internal and external forces are linked together. The Five Great Elements are:

Earth, the solid state of matter, whose characteristic attribute is stability, fixity or rigidity. Earth is stable substance.

Water, the liquid state of matter, whose characteristic attribute is flux. Water is substance without stability.

Fire, the power that can convert a substance from solid to liquid to gas or vice versa, increasing or decreasing the substance's relative order. Fire is form without substance; its characteristic attribute is transformation.

Air, the gaseous state of matter, whose characteristic attribute is mobility or dynamism. Air is existence without form.

Space, the *field* from which everything is manifested and into which everything returns; the space in which events occur. Space (which can also be translated "Ether") has no physical existence; it exists only as the distances that separate matter.

The Three Doshas

These Five Elements condense to the Three Doshas: Vata, Pitta and Kapha. Vata, Pitta and Kapha are effectively Air, Fire and Water respectively. Vata, which is the principle of kinetic energy in the body, is mainly concerned with the nervous system, and controls all body movement. Kapha, the principle of potential energy, controls body stability and lubrication. The tissues and wastes of the body, which Vata moves around, are Kapha's province. Pitta controls the body's balance of kinetic and potential energies. All of Pitta's processes involve digestion or "cooking," even if it is the cooking of thoughts into theories in the mind. The enzymatic and endocrine systems are Pitta's main field of activity.

At the cellular level Vata moves nutrients into and wastes out of cells, Pitta digests nutrients to provide energy for cellular function, and Kapha governs the cell's structure. In the digestive tract Vata chews and swallows the food, Pitta digests it, Vata assimilates nutrients and expels wastes, and Kapha controls the secretions that lubricate and protect the digestive organs. In the mind Vata retrieves previous data from memory for comparison with new data. Pitta processes the new data and draws conclusions, which Vata then stores as new memories. Kapha provides the stability needed for the mind to grasp a single thought at a time.

These three are forces, not substances. Kapha is not mucus; it is the force which when projected into the body causes mucus to arise. Pitta is not bile; it is the force that causes bile to be produced. Vata is not gas, but increased Vata increases gas. Vata, Pitta and Kapha are called doshas because the word *dosha* means "a thing that can go out of whack." When Vata, Pitta and Kapha are out of balance with one another the system is bound to lose its own balance.

Kapha, the Watery Dosha, is associated with Water and Earth, two Elements that have no real affinity for one another. When you pour sand into water, for example, it drops to the bottom of the vessel and sits there. No matter how hard you try to get them to interact on their own the sand will remain suspended in the water only so long as you continue to stir it. Kapha forces Water and Earth, which would otherwise refuse to interact with one another, to combine properly and remain in a mutually satisfying equilibrium.

Nature has provided us with Kapha to keep the body's Earth (its solids) suspended in its Water (its liquids) in the proper proportion. Wherever the body becomes too solid a problem always develops. Gall stones and kidney stones are good examples of concretions of Earth in which Water has dried out too much to let free flow continue. Likewise, too much Water and not enough Earth in a system promotes disturbances like edema. Only when Kapha is balanced do Water and Earth remain in balance.

Pitta, the Fiery Element, is associated with both Fire and Water. While Water and Earth would love to be able to ignore one another and are inert to each other when they do mix, Fire and Water are always antagonistic. Mix Fire and Water together and the one or the other is bound to come out uppermost. When Fire is stronger than Water it will boil off or evaporate Water, and even boiling Water can overpower and drown out a Fire in sufficient quantitiy. To make two such opponents cooperate is Pitta's job.

All "fires" in the body are contained in water. Stomach acid is for instance an extremely powerful acid, with a pH of 2. It burns anything it touches as surely as open flame or a bolt of lightning will burn. Acid is Fire contained in Water.

When Fire predominates in this mixture the acid can burn through the natural containment facilities that Water provides. If this happens in the stomach a gastric ulcer will result. Should Water predominate it will douse the Fire and create indigestion. Only the mediation that healthy Pitta provides can keep this uneasy alliance of Fire and Water intact.

Air and Space compose Vata. Air, like wind in the external universe, can move freely in the body only when its path is free of obstacles. You are safe from strong wind in your home, unless the wind happens to be so strong that it blows down your walls. Likewise, insufficient empty space in the form of the Space Element prevents proper movement of Air, unless Air's force accumulates sufficiently to blast a free passage for itself.

Space is totally inert; Air is totally mobile. Air always attempts to expand itself free from limitations. If this expansive tendency becomes too pronounced it will destroy any structure that limits it, creating for example the spontaneous fractures that happen to hip joints that have been weakened by osteoporosis. When excessive empty space and insufficient power of movement combine stasis can result. Emphysema is one example of such a condition; another is the type of constipation that develops after overuse of enemas or colonics. Only healthy Vata can keep Air and Space balanced with one another, by ensuring that there is just sufficient Space for Air to move in and just enough Air to move within it.

Ayurveda is fundamentally a qualitative medical system. Everything in the universe that is external to us affects its counterparts within us by means of its inherent qualities. The qualities that characterize every substance we consume and every action we perform also serve either to reinforce or to attenuate the natural qualities, or attributes, of the Three Doshas. These characteristics are:

Vata	Pitta	Kapha
dry	oily	oily
cold	**hot**	cold
light	light	**heavy**
irregular	intense	stable
mobile	fluid	viscous
rarefied	malodorous	dense
rough	liquid	smooth

Vata possesses all the qualities we usually associate with air. It dries, just as even a mild, moist breeze eventually dries clothes hung on a line. It cools, just as even a hot wind can cool a body by evaporating sweat from its skin. It roughens, just as the desert wind erodes the mesas and buttes of the desert. It is erratic, or irregular, advancing usually in puffs and gusts rather than a steady stream. Wind is not rough in itself, nor need it be dry or cold to cause dryness or coldness. Its innate effects take precedence over the conditional qualities it picks up from its environment.

Pitta likewise produces its effects because of its own innate characteristics. It is oily, or unctuous, not because fire is oily but because oils and fats burn brightly in fire. Like fire it is hot, intense, and light, and its fluidity and liquidity derive from the fact that it is Fire contained in Water. Because it is fluid and can engulf and devour food it is able to digest and transform.

Kapha has all the same qualities as mucus. It is viscid, which makes it slow moving. It is also cold, heavy, dull, thick, smooth, sticky, and sluggish, all qualities which we associate with mud, a substance composed of Earth suspended in Water. Yogurt is a characteristic example of a Kapha-type food because it too possesses all these attributes.

Note that:

Both Pitta and Kapha are oily, and Vata is dry, so *dryness* is characteristic of Vata. Dryness appears in the body or mind only when there is increase of Vata.

Dryness is a side-effect of *motion*, which is Vata's physiological function. The *unevenness* of excessive dryness introduces *irregularity* into the body and mind.

Both Vata and Kapha are cold, and Pitta is hot, so heat is characteristic of Pitta. *Heat* appears in the body or mind only when there is disturbance of Pitta.

Heat is aside-effect of *transformation*, which is Pitta's physiological function. The *intensity* of excessive heat introduces *irritability* into the body and mind.

Both Vata and Pitta are light, and Kapha is heavy, so *heaviness* is characteristic of Kapha. Heaviness appears in the body or mind only when there is disturbance of Kapha.

Heaviness is a side-effect of *stability*, which is Kapha's physiological function. The *viscosity* of excessive heaviness introduces *slowness* into the body and mind.

Vata, Pitta and Kapha all possess their own unique inherent qualities, and they enjoy distinctive affinities for certain bodily organs. They are all present in each cell, since they are essential to life, but they tend to congregate in certain areas:

Vata	Pitta	Kapha
Brain	Skin	Brain
Heart	Eyes	Joints
Colon	Liver	Mouth
Bones	Brain	Lymph
Lungs	Blood	Stomach
Bladder	Spleen	Pleural Cavity
Bone Marrow	Endocrine	Pericardial Cavity
Nervous System	Small Intestine	

Vata and Kapha are almost totally opposite one another in quality. Kapha, which represents all potential states of energy in the body, permits energy to be stored. Vata, which represents all kinetic states of energy in the body, causes stored energy to be released. Vata promotes change, but excessive change can lead to overstimulation. Kapha promotes stasis, but excessive stasis can lead to inertia. Pitta is in charge of balancing these two diametrically contrary forces.

Vata and Kapha congregate near one another for practical reasons. The heart and lungs are continuously in motion and so require continuous lubrication. Vata provides the motion, Kapha the lubrication. Too much motion uses up the lubricant; too much lubricant gums up the works. In the joints, synovial fluid provides lubrication and protection. The brain and spinal cord, whose movement is confined to nerve impulses, swim in cerebrospinal fluid. Mucus protects the lining of the gut throughout its length, enabling the food within it to pass freely. Movement and stability, and the force that balances them: Vata, Kapha and Pitta.

Vata, Pitta and Kapha are together essential to life, and can cause great harm if they are allowed to fall out of harmony with one another. Their personalities are two-faced because they are doshas, things that are often in error. This is not really their fault because they have such thankless jobs to do. Kapha must overcome the mutual indifference of Water and Earth and make them work together, Pitta must conquer the natural animosity which Water and Fire feel for one another, and Vata is forced to use the inert Space to try to control the capricious Air. Given the difficulty of these tasks it is quite surprising that they function as well as they do.

Because they are so reactive the body cannot afford to store the Three Doshas within itself for long, any more than a nuclear power plant can afford to store radioactive wastes on its premises. The Three Doshas are therefore eliminated from the body regularly in the course of performing their functions. The force of Kapha is continually expelled from the body via mucus, Pitta is regularly excreted through acid and bile, and Vata is eliminated both as gas and as muscular or nervous energy.

The Six Tastes

Regular elimination of the Doshas is so essential because our normal metabolic processes continuously produce them. How much of each Dosha your body produces depends primarily on which of the Six Tastes you consume. The Six Tastes, which like the Three Doshas are derived from the Five Great Elements, help to mediate the balance of the body's doshas by performing essential functions for the organism. The Tastes, which are capitalized here to emphasize the profound effect they have not merely on the tongue but on all parts of the organism, are Sweet, Sour, Salty, Pungent, Bitter and Astringent.

> **Sweet** - Composed mainly of Earth and Water, Sweet increases Kapha, decreases Pitta and Vata, and is cooling, heavy and unctuous. It nourishes and exhilarates the body and mind and relieves hunger and thirst.

It promotes increase in all tissues.

Sour - Composed mainly of Earth and Fire, Sour increases Kapha and Pitta, decreases Vata, and is heating, heavy and unctuous. Sour refreshes the being, encourages elimination of wastes, encourages spasms and tremors to abate, and improves appetite and digestion.

Salty - Composed mainly of Water and Fire, Salty increases Kapha and Pitta, decreases Vata, and is heavy, heating and unctuous. Salty eliminates wastes, cleanses the body and increases the digestive capacity and appetite. It softens and loosens the tissues.

Pungent - Composed mainly of Fire and Air, Pungent (which is hot and spicy like chili peppers) increases Pitta and Vata, decreases Kapha, and is heating, light, and dry. Pungent flushes all types of secretions from the body and diminishes all Kapha-like tissues such as semen, milk and fat. It improves the appetite.

Bitter - Composed mainly of Air and Space, Bitter increases Vata, decreases Pitta and Kapha, and is cooling, light and dry. Bitter purifies and dries all secretions, is anti-aphrodisiac, and tones the organism by returning all Tastes to normal balance. It amplifies appetite and restrains skin diseases and fevers.

Astringent - Composed mainly of Air and Earth, Astringent (which makes your mouth pucker) increases Vata, decreases Pitta and Kapha, and is cooling, light and dry. Astringent heals, purifies and constricts all parts of the body. It reduces all secretions and is anti-aphrodisiac.

All Six of the Tastes are essential for proper functioning of the organism and reach us primarily through our food. My teacher Vimalananda always maintained that it's not what you eat but what you digest that counts. The healthiest food in the world will become for you the deadliest of poisons if you cannot digest and assimilate it properly. Digestion begins in the mouth at the instant the tongue Tastes the food, for by the time the food reaches the gut the digestive organs must be ready for it. The tongue transmits the food's Tastes directly to the brain, which determines from this testimony what sort of fat, protein or carbohydrate has been ingested and what sort of juices need to be secreted for optimal digestion.

Diners who praise delicious dishes misdirect their praise, because Taste is really present in the mouth, not in the food. A food that is described as Sweet, for example, is a food that is experienced as Sweet by most healthy individuals under ordinary conditions. A good-quality orange tastes both Sweet and Sour to a normal human tongue, but the condition of your internal Tastes may sometimes make you taste it as Sweeter and sometimes as more Sour.

As an experiment, cut an orange into two halves and eat one half. Then take a teaspoonful of something Sweet, like honey or maple syrup, and finally eat the other half of the orange. No matter how Sweet the first half seemed, the orange's second half will Taste less Sweet, more Sour. What has changed is your sense of Taste, not the orange. The sweetener you took temporarily satiated your body's capacity for Sweet. When the second half of the orange entered your mouth your tongue ignored the Taste it had plenty of and selectively experienced Sour, the orange's other Taste.

Another example of the internal nature of Taste utilizes a leaf from India known as *madhuvinashini*, which translates as "Killer of Sweet." Madhuvinashini (*Gymnema sylvestre*; in Hindi, gurmar) temporarily abolishes the Sweet Taste when chewed. Even after a small quantity of the leaf sugar loses its Sweetness, and your tongue experiences only its texture rather than its Taste. Since sugar's sole Taste is Sweet, it becomes just like soluble sand. Apples retain their Sourness even after the Sweet is gone; licorice root loses its Sweetness but retains most of its Bitterness. Some Bitterness is lost because this leaf also reduces Bitter slightly. Sweet and Bitter are two sides of the same coin.

Taste does not disappear from food even after it is digested. Each of your cells has a rudimentary sense of Taste, and each is affected by the Taste of its nutrients. Since each cell in your body affects every other cell, and since all those cells affect your senses and your mind, the Tastes in the food you eat exert a critical influence on your consciousness and your health. Taste predominates over all other physical influences on the individual, even the doshas, because taste is the first input from ingested food that the system receives.

Everything you eat has three opportunities to affect your organism:

The effect a food has on you *before digestion* begins is the taste your tongue picks up from it while it is in the mouth. This effect is called *Rasa*, or *Taste*.

The second effect, which is experienced *during digestion*, is the food's *Virya*, or *Energy*. "Hot" food increases the body's ability to digest, freeing energy for other metabolic tasks. "Cold" food requires extra energy for its digestion. The gut obtains this energy from the rest of the body, which must reduce its other activities as a result.

The *Vipaka*, or *Post-Digestive Effect* is that which occurs after digestion is over and the nutrients are assimilated deep within the tissues. Sweet and Salty usually produce a Sweet, satisfying, nutritive effect after being digested, a net gain for your organism. Sour usually produces a Sour effect, increasing the desire for new things to digest but neither adding to nor subtracting much from you. Bitter, Pungent and Astringent generally produce Pungency, which causes things, physical and mental, to be consumed or to flow out of you. The Bitter and Astringent Tastes reduce Pitta because their cold Taste and Energy more than compensate for the Pungency that their Post-Digestive Effect usually produces.

TasteEnergy		Post-Digestive
Sweet	Cold	Sweet
Sour	Hot	Sour
Salty	Hot	Sweet
Pungent	Hot	Pungent
Bitter	Cold	Pungent
Astringent	Cold	Pungent

Sour, Salty and Pungent are always "hot," and Sweet, Bitter and Astringent are always "cold." Some substances may however possess both a heating Taste and Cold Energy, which means that it will increase the digestive power when it enters the body but will not during digestion aggravate Pitta. Some substances are organized the other way round, with a cooling Taste and Hot Energy. These reduce appetite when eaten but increase digestive juice flow while digestion is going on.

Cooked onions are Sweet in Taste, Hot in Energy, and Sweet in Post-Digestive Effect. They satisfy hunger with their Sweet Taste and promote anabolism with their Sweet Post-Digestive Effect, but their Hot Energy prevents their Sweetness from disturbing Kapha.

Lemons are Sour, Bitter and Astringent in Taste, Cold in Energy, and Sweet in Post-Digestive Effect. Being Bitter they tone the body and prevent Kapha increase, being Sour they increase digestion and appetite and relieve Vata. Their Cold Energy prevents Pitta from being disturbed, and their Sweet Post-Digestive Effect means they assist in tissue nutrition. Those substances that most effectively balance the organism are usually those that are most unique in their pattern of qualities.

EFFECTS OF OVERUSE

You can maintain balance among the Six Tastes as long as you do not persist in overusing one or more of them. The effects of overuse of specific Tastes include:

Sweet - obesity, diabetes, dropsy, parasites, obstructed circulation, eye inflammation, indigestion, vomiting, gas, lethargy, respiratory congestion and other Kapha-type disturbances.

Sour - burning sensations, itches, giddiness, premature aging and looseness of body tissues, suppuration.

Salty - inflammation, edema, easy bleeding, skin diseases including herpes and hives, joint disease, impotence, early wrinkling of the skin, early baldness.

Pungent - pain, dizziness, loss of consciousness, dryness of the mouth, tremors, debility, emaciation, burning sensations, fever, increased thirst, drying of sexual secretions.

Bitter - all Vata diseases including numbness, emaciation, cutting or breaking or colicky pain, giddiness, headache, stiffness, tremors, decreased sexual secretions.

Astringent - all types of Vata disturbance including tremors, fits, constipation, dryness of the body, distention, tingling numbness, emaciation, thirst, decreased sexual secretions.

The relative intensity of the Tastes in a food determines that food's effects on the Three Doshas. Salty is most effective among the Vata-controlling Tastes because it is heavy, oily and heating, and it improves digestion. Sour comes next and then Sweet. Bitter is the best Pitta-controlling Taste because it is cooling and drying. Sweet comes next and then Astringent. Pungent best controls Kapha because it is heating, light and dry and it flushes secretions from the body. Bitter comes next and then Astringent.

Two of the first signs of disturbance in body tissues are the mistaking of one Taste for another and the inability to experience Taste at all. Both these conditions usually result from the overuse of one or more Tastes. This dullness of the Taste sense makes it impossible for the brain to properly prepare the body for the incoming food, which in turn prevents proper digestion.

The Six Tastes are even more important to the mind than they are to the body, thanks to the mind's craving for sensory stimulation. The mind employs two groups of senses: the five senses of perception, which we all know well, and the five senses of action. The five action senses are the voice (which symbolizes all forms of communication), hands (which symbolize manipulation of all types), feet (locomotion), genitals (creation and procreation) and anus (elimination).

Each sense of perception is a channel through which the mind moves to a sense object, experiences it, and returns to process its experience. Each sense of action is a channel into which the mind enters in order to express itself by projecting its personality into the outside world, and through which it returns again after completing its expression.

Sensory channels can, like any other channel, suffer from an excess of either dilation or constriction. Overuse of a sense organ overdilates its channel, enervating that sense so that the mind can no longer obtain enjoyment from its use. Underuse of a sense constricts that sense organ's channel, which also reduces the mind's ability to enjoy itself along that pathway. An overdilated channel provides too much Space for Air to move properly in; an overconstricted channel is an obstruction to Air's unimpeded movement. Overuse, underuse, misuse and abuse of the sense organs are collectively regarded in Ayurveda as one of the three main causes of human disease.

PREDOMINANT EMOTIONS

The most significant among the many factors that influence the dilation and constriction of the sensory channels are probably Taste and emotion. The Sanskrit word rasa means, among other things, both "taste" and "emotion."

This suggests that Taste and emotion are identical forces on different planes of existence, that Taste is to the body what emotion is to the mind. An emotion that appears in the mind tends to produce in the body its corresponding Taste, just as a Taste when ingested tends to create in the mind its corresponding emotion. The predominant attitudes and emotions associated with the Tastes are:

Sweet - satisfaction, or satiation (the "sweet taste of success"). Overindulgence in Sweet leads to its negative aspects: complacency and greed.

Sour - the searching outside oneself for things to possess. Sour enhances the mind's appetite for evaluating things with a view to determining their desirability as possessions. Overindulgence in evaluation leads to envy or jealousy, which may manifest as deprecation of the thing desired, as in the "sour grapes" syndrome.

Salty - zest for life, which enhances all appetites. Overindulgence in zest leads to hedonism, the craving for indulgence in all sensory pleasures that are available, just as an "old salt" or a "salty dog" will do when he enters port again after a long sea voyage.

Pungent - extroversion, the tendency to excitement and stimulation, and in particular the craving for intensity. Overexcitement and overstimulation lead to irritability, impatience and anger ("pungent language," "a sharp retort").

Bitter - dissatisfaction, which produces a desire to change. When you have to swallow a "bitter pill" its bitterness dispels your self-delusion and forces you to face reality. Too much disappointment leads to frustration, which confirms your system in bitterness. Grief is Bitter.

Astringent - introversion, which drags the mind away from excitement and stimulation. Excessive introversion leads to insecurity, anxiety and fear. Astringency causes contraction, which makes you "shrivel like a prune," and clamps the "cold, bony hand of fear" around your throat.

At all times your personality tries to maintain itself in the greatest possible comfort. It seeks the satisfaction of Sweet, and will make use of any other Taste it requires to obtain it, selecting "hot" or "cold" Tastes according to its requirements. Sour, Salty and Pungent are "hot" Tastes and Sweet, Bitter and Astringent are "cold" Tastes. Each of their corresponding emotions is accordingly hot or cold. Heat expands and cold contracts, in health as in physics. Cold constricts physical and mental channels, and heat dilates them.

Sweet, Bitter and Astringent are cooling Tastes, and their corresponding emotions are cold and contracting. They decrease the organism's desire to "eat" new things. Satisfaction or complacency is a constricting emotion because it lessens the mind's appetite for enjoyment through a sense. Dissatisfaction constricts because it is an admission of inability to enjoy through a sense. Fear, the most powerful of all constricting emotions, constricts all senses. Fear actually produces constriction in the bronchioles of susceptible individuals and can initiate asthmatic attacks.

Sour, Salty and Pungent are hot Tastes, and their corresponding emotions are hot and expansive. They increase the organism's desire to consume food or other sense objects. This is hedonism, Salty's emotion. Envy or jealousy actively increases the mind's desire to enjoy. Anger indirectly increases the physical and mental appetites by flooding the organism with heat.

Salty is called "all-tastes" (*sarva rasa* in Sanskrit) because it can enhance all flavors in a food while simultaneously increasing the organism's appetite for food. It promotes good digestion when used in small amounts as a condiment, and weakens the body when used in excess. "Hedonism," the emotion associated with Salty, does the same for the mind: while small amounts increase the mind's desire for intensity of experience, overuse makes the mind vapid and weak.

Salty forces the body to retain water and increases the production of digestive juices and sexual fluids, which is why salt is contraindicated in those who wish to remain celibate. In fact, Salty increases all body juices. Life itself is based in water—each of us is 75% water—so more juices make for a "juicier" life. When powerfully impelled by the Salty Taste to gratify themselves, your senses will force you to immerse yourself in worldly pursuits. Salt and the Salty Taste are intoxicants, literally, and like all other intoxicants they possess a potential for abuse.

EFFECTS ON CONSCIOUSNESS

Actually all Tastes can be used as intoxicants. Sweet, for example, is a popular drug in our society; people use it to feel satisfied. Some societies intoxicate themselves with the envy of Sour or the irritability of Pungent, and some individuals may even use Bitter and Astringent for self-gratification. We all use our food to alter our consciousness, and all alterations of consciousness affect the body via the Three Doshas:

Sweet's intense complacent effect increases the naturally inert, complacent Kapha, cools the anger of Pitta and comforts the fear of Vata.

Sour's envious effect increases Kapha when envy of another's success incites you to clutch all the more firmly to your own belongings. Otherwise Pitta will increase as jealousy mutates into anger over the raw deal you feel you are getting from life. Envy can help reduce your Vata by focusing and heating up your consciousness.

Salty's "hedonism" increases complacency as long as you are able to indulge, which increases Kapha. It increases the fieriness of Pitta's anger whenever there is any obstruction to your gratification, and decreases Vata by allaying fears of inadequacy or inability to properly indulge.

Pungent increases Pitta by actively increasing the flow of hormones and digestive juices, making it easier both to digest and to manifest anger. It relieves Kapha by decreasing self-satisfaction, and temporarily relieves

Vata by facilitating expression of bottled-up emotions. In the long run, however, Pungent increases Vata by exhausting the organs and glands. This "dries you out," limiting your ability to project aggression or unhappiness outwards.

Bitter is the best of all Six Tastes. As Dr. Vasant Lad likes to say, "Bitter is better." In small amounts Bitter helps balance all other tastes in the body. In the same way that mild dissatisfaction with yourself or your situation impels you to change, Bitter dilates channels that are too constricted (thus reducing Kapha and its complacency) and constricts those which are too dilated (thus reducing Pitta and its anger). Overuse of Bitter increases Vata, as dissatisfaction and continuous change induce insecurity and fear.

Astringent constricts, drawing one away from the self-satisfaction of Kapha and the self-aggrandizement of Pitta. Its constriction increases fear of insufficient sensory "nutrition" and leads to increased Vata.

Bitter, Pungent and Astringent all increase Vata and decrease Kapha. Their lightness reduces your desire to remain connected with your body, and makes it more difficult for your personality to self-identify with your body even if it wants to continue to do so. Sweet, Sour and Salty all increase Kapha and decrease Vata. Their heaviness enhances both your ability to self-identify with your body and your interest in doing so. We are all prey to our Tastes and emotions.

For example, we live in a consumer culture. In order for our economy to continue to function we are all expected to go deeply into debt. To promote spending Madison Avenue through its advertising wizardry brings into being within us new desires for things we never before had and usually do not need. First the desire for a hedonistic lifestyle is created, which creates the Salty Taste within us. Next comes envy, as we compare ourselves to the Jones's next door and realize how much more and better they are able to gratify their senses than are we. This produces the Sour Taste. Finally, our impatience to be able to gratify ourselves manifests as anger when some obstacle comes in our way; this creates Pungent.

Salty, Sour and Pungent being Hot Tastes we are now "all heated up," ready to consume and digest, physically and mentally. All remains well as long as we are able to obtain enough "food" (for any of our senses) to satisfy this hunger. Inevitably, however, some of these created desires remain unfulfilled. Even with unlimited wealth at your disposal there are a limited number of hours in the day. How much can you spend? How much can you gratify yourself? Your unfulfilled desires are likely to create Bitterness within you if they lead you into dissatisfaction.

Ayurveda teaches us that the Bitter Taste is in small doses a tonic for the appetite and digestion. It works this way in the world as well, for a little dissatisfaction can spur you on to greater and greater appetites. Too much dissatisfaction though and you will end up with an excess of Bitterness in your organism. When you don't have sufficient energy—money—to go around you will have to prioritize your indulgences, which will lead to frustration at being unable to achieve the state of constantly repeated enjoyment that the media projects at you ceaselessly. Excessive Bitterness overstimulates Vata and disturbs your mind as you brood over your state.

Sour, Salty and Pungent perfuse your being while you have the interest and ability to indulge, and, once your indulgence is interrupted, Bitter floods your organism. Your body knows it has a Taste imbalance, and knows that Sweet can be used to rebalance the situation, so it craves Sweet. Sweet satisfies the hungers generated by Sour, Salty and Pungent, and being Bitter's exact opposite it eliminates frustration and dissatisfaction. Once Sweet is consumed the body and mind temporarily return to balance and feel pleased with themselves.

The mind does not have to consume food in order to obtain Sweetness. It can derive Sweet from any thrill-producing activity, even a shopping spree. The temporary sensation of unlimited power inherent in a credit card provides powerful gratification, which unfortunately disappears almost as soon as the purchaser returns home with the purchases.

Well-digested food satisfies longer than other thrills can because, even after the initial rush of pleasure is gone, properly digested and assimilated food will be nourishing and gratifying thousands of body cells. Unsatisfactory digestion creates the same secondary dissatisfaction that results from any other cheap thrill; it flatters only to deceive. The tissues are momentarily taken in by the promise of substantial nutrition, and feel jilted when the smoke clears and the sensation is gone.

Even when there is good digestion, the intensity of the Sweet sensation abates as soon as the food has been digested and assimilated. The tendency then is to eat again, to experience again the temporary somatic bliss which food affords. This tendency is even more pronounced if digestion is poor, because despite food intake little nutrition actually reaches the tissues, which then send messages to the mind to remind it that they are starving. The more you eat in such a condition the weaker your digestion will become.

Soon the individual begins to crave Sour, Salty and Pungent as well as Sweet because the "hot" Tastes enkindle the digestive fires to request further gratification by food. Sour, Salty and Pungent also enhance the appetite, however, so no matter how much you eat you will always be hungry for more.

Fast food, which now accounts for half of all meals served in the U.S.A., developed because the cravings for immediate gratification of the tongue that may arise at any moment must be speedily slaked. Think of French fries: the potatoes, which are Sweet, are served with a thick frosting of Salt and slathered in Sweet-Sour-Salty ketchup. The eater gets his or her Sweet fix with sufficient Sour and Salty to awaken the taste buds and the digestive organs. Or the noble hamburger: Sweet-Sour mayonnaise plus Sour-Salty-Pungent mustard plus Sweet-Sour-Salty pickles all on a Sweet wheaten bun. And the taco, which has all these Tastes plus an increased quantity of Pungent to further stimulate an already overstimulated digestive tract.

Junk "foods," which are junk because they are all taste and no nutrition, are usually washed down with soft drinks or coffee. Most soft drinks are intensely Sweet, and many have the added bonus of caffeine. Coffee is Pungent, plus whatever Sweet is added with cream and sugar, and is also full of caffeine. Caffeine is a metabolic credit card, a substance which forces the body to secrete enough hormones to keep us functioning, gratifying ourselves with Sweetness in its various forms until we drop from fatigue. Like the fiscal debt we are encouraged to create, most of us develop crushing burdens of physiological debt by use of such "credit cards."

Eventually all the bills come due. Unlike financial institutions and Third World countries your organism cannot default on its debts, except by dying. Perhaps diabetes develops, a disease in which the body can no longer cope with the tremendous quantities of Sweet which the mind requires, and begins to discard it undigested. Or maybe your thyroid or adrenals collapse from their debt burden and your system goes on a general strike.

Your personal constitution, which is your individual metabolic makeup, helps determine how much effect specific tastes and emotions are likely have on you. This is why everyone who eats the same food does not necessarily experience exactly the same mental or physical effects from it. When all the members of a family enjoy a meal together, each individual's tastes and emotions will be affected according to his or her individual taste and emotional balance.

Your inborn metabolic pattern is called *prakriti*. Prakriti also means Nature, She who is the first creation. Your prakriti is your first "creation," your first reaction when you are forced to adapt to some change in your environment. Your constitution is that set of metabolic tendencies which determine how your body and mind will instinctively react when they are confronted by a stimulus. Many of the traits you prize in your personality arise from and are dependent on these metabolic tendencies. Many of the qualities you dislike in yourself also arise from these tendencies. Knowing your constitution allows you to know your body and mind better. You learn why there is no need to feel guilty for your dietary preferences, or for your mental traits like anger or fear. Once you understand that these traits are determined by your constitution, lifestyle changes can help your organism minimize their influence.

Your personal constitution was determined by the state of the bodies of your mother and father at the time of your conception. That certain sperm which could best endure the conditions prevalent in those two bodies won the race to reach the ovum and its genes mingled with the genes in the ovum to form the new child. Your constitution is influenced by your parents' genetics, by your mother's diet and habits during her pregnancy, and by any abnormal events at the time of your birth. Once your personal constitution and its accompanying tendencies have been set they cannot be permanently altered. You have both your genes and your constitution for the rest of your life, like them or not.

You can, however, learn to adjust for your constitution so that you are less affected by its distortions. You can learn how to prevent health imbalances and how to best treat them when they arise. You can know the prognosis of any disease you might contract, and you can determine which rejuvenation program will be best for you. Through study and use of Ayurvedic principles you can also understand why your spouse, children, relatives, friends, neighbors and co-workers do the things they do, and determine how best to interact with them for maximum interpersonal harmony. You can plan meals for your family according to what is best for each of their prakritis.

Ayurveda is a very common-sense sort of medical system. It uses very simple, easy-to-understand principles to determine individual prakriti. Because these principles are based in the theory of the Three Doshas your prakriti is expressed in terms of Vata, Pitta and Kapha. Vata-type people actually are more Airy and Ethereal than are other people. Their bodies tend to produce more intestinal gas, and their minds tend to be more "spacey." Even the crackling noise their joints make is said by some authorities to be due to the displacement of bubbles of nitrogen in those joints. Pitta-type people literally have more Fire in them than do other types. They have better appetites and better digestion, can withstand cold better, and are more hotheaded. Kapha people tend to have heavier, earthier bodies than do other types, and tend to store Watery substances like fluids and fat more readily than do others. Ayurveda looks at individuals through the lenses of Vata, Pitta and Kapha.

Your constitution also influences your emotions. For example, if you have a constitutional tendency to Vata increase you will be anxious and fearful by nature. You will naturally crave Sweet, Sour and Salty, which reduce Vata and thus assuage fear. However, if you try to feel better and better by overeating Sweet, Sour and Salty you will increase Kapha, which can obstruct the free movement of Vata and produce disease. Vata people who wish to be healthy should eat mainly Sweet, Sour and Salty foods in amounts small enough to be easily digested.

People who are mainly Kapha constitutionally sometimes use Sweet, Sour and Salty to further entrench themselves in their set ways, when they should be using the Bitter, Pungent and Astringent Tastes to shake up and awaken themselves. It is not possible to stay alive on Bitter, Pungent and Astringent alone, but these Tastes should form a significant portion of the diet.

People who have Pitta-type constitutions are naturally aggressive and impatient. Sweet, Bitter and Astringent are the best tastes to combat this innate tendency and promote balance. Unfortunately Pitta-type people frequently choose Sour, Salty and Pungent food, which makes them even more aggressive, impatient and ruthless, and revs them up for greater and greater achievement, which is a hallmark of the Pitta personality. Such food tends to overheat their bodies and minds, however, and leads to imbalance.

Your constitution affects your emotions, and the Tastes you crave, via your genes. Scientists have already located genes that influence a variety of the emotional states that flesh is heir to. Each emotion is not likely to be controlled by a single gene, but since all mental states have a physical basis there is bound to be somewhere in your genome a pattern of genes which produce a set of proteins which interact with a bevy of hormones to produce the physical state that induces the expression of the emotion. And vice versa—your emotions can trigger certain of your genes to work and others to remain dormant, thus affecting your hormones and your metabolic balance.

If your parents and grandparents were easily angered there is a strong likelihood that they will pass down to you a gene or a set of genes that will make you prone to anger easily. If they were fearful you will probably inherit fear genes which may promote a lifelong tendency to be dogged by fear. Each of us lives in an emotional ocean spawned from our genes.

Though our genes are activated and deactivated by the Tastes we ingest they do not directly change under the influence of these Tastes. Frequently used genes may become easier to activate and rarely used genes may recede from view, but all our genes continue to lie in wait for an opportunity to display themselves so long as we live. And, as long as your genes exist your tendency to certain emotions will stay with you. Until you can change your genes you will have to rely on knowing your own personal constitution if you hope to bring yourself into balance. Understanding your prakriti gives you insight into why you do the things you do, and can give you clues on how to improve yourself.

Chapter Two
Constitutional Characteristics

There are eight possible constitutional types:
V, P, K, VP, PK, VK, VPK and Balanced.

The small number of VPK individuals whose three dosha energies are constitutionally out of balance are rarely healthy and must live a very disciplined life to remain disease free. Members of the smaller group of constitutionally balanced individuals usually remain healthy, for they must be severely stressed before an imbalance develops. We will concentrate here on the other six types, who form the great majority of people. For convenience Vata has been abbreviated to V, Pitta to P and Kapha to K.

To determine your own individual constitution you will need to evaluate yourself as accurately and as honestly as you can. Avoid the temptation to see yourself as you would like to be rather than as you are. You will be wise to have a friend or family member evaluate you as well and then compare the two evaluations to ensure clarity. There is no right or wrong, and no better or worse, in this examination. There is only the reality of your personal constitution. Everyone passes who answers this exam honestly, and everyone fails who doctors their answers to make them conform more closely to their perceived self-image. Like them or not your constitutional proclivities are yours, and like mooching kinfolk they will stick with you as long as you live. You may as well learn to live with them, and learn how to change your life so that you maximize your possibilities for health.

Please respond below according to how you have reacted in general throughout your entire lifetime, not how you react at present. Select the description which fits you most perfectly overall. If in any category there have been great changes at various times in your life please select Vata as your answer even if the Vata description in that category does not accurately describe you as you are today. For example, if you have had wide fluctuations in your weight all during your life, so that you were significantly overweight at certain periods and almost underweight at others, you should answer "Vata" for your weight even if you are overweight at present.

Most people are not purely Vata or Pitta or Kapha in nature; most fit predominantly into one category and secondarily into another. Their constitution is derived from the conditions of the bodies of both their parents at the time of their conception. Unless both parents were very close to one another in body type and health the variation between them at that moment will show up as a variation in your constitution. This is why most people have dual constitutions and why it may not always be easy to know which force predominates in you.

Fortunately, some characteristics are ordinarily quite reliable. Narrow shoulders and/or hips almost always appear in V people, and broad shoulders and/or hips are almost always characteristic of Kapha. People whose skins are dark or who tan easily usually have a lot of Vata, while those who cannot tan at all or tan very little are ordinarily very Pitta, especially if their hair is fine.

If in any one category you feel that you belong partly in one constitution and partly in another, write down both. If in any one category you feel you might fit into all three constitutions select the two which best characterize you. Whenever there is significant doubt or confusion, select "Vata."

While evaluating yourself, keep in mind that:

Vata is cold, dry and irregular.
Pitta is hot, oily and irritable.
Kapha is cold, wet and stable.

Each constitutional type has its own inborn approach to managing its physical and mental energies, and each possesses an innate strategy for dealing with situations in which it is called upon to adapt. That Vata is governed by kinetic energy, the energy of action, inspires V people make active use of their energy. They spend freely and frequently waste their energies because of this predilection for action. K types, who are governed by the potential energy of Kapha, have a decided tendency to store energy within themselves. They have a genetic predisposition to save and supervise energy well. Pitta is in charge of balancing and managing Vata and Kapha, and P people are born experts in efficiently managing and using energies of all sorts. Whether engaged in exercise, money making, speaking, sex, or even sleeping and dreaming an individual's innate pattern of energy utilization depends upon his or her prakriti.

Vata exerts a cold, dry, irregular influence on the system because as soon as energy enters the organism it is expended, leaving emptiness behind. Kapha has a cold, wet, stable influence and a K-type person is rarely empty because most of the energy that enters the individual remains stored within. Pitta's effect is hot, oily and irritable because Pitta must maintain a high level of reactivity in order to manipulate energy effectively.

Each of the categories below will help illustrate to you the approach that your system follows in its own energy utilization. The evaluation criteria may seem complex because of the difficulty in describing in words concepts which are easy to see but hard to explain. If you feel confused by the difficult categories ignore them and pay more attention to the easier ones. Remember that Ayurveda is based in common sense, and rely on your own common sense to understand and use it.

Prakriti Evaluation

BODY FRAME
V people tend to be either unusually tall or unusually short. They grow like weeds and most often remain slender or rangy, with a thin body frame and

narrow shoulders and/or hips. Their arms or legs may seem unusually short or, more often, unusually long. They tend to have long, tapering fingers and toes. Any significant departure from any body proportion is usually due to Vata, via Vata's quality of *irregularity.*

V people may have very light, small bones, or heavy bones with joints that are prominent or protrude. Their joints tend to make cracking noises when they move. If you show most of these characteristics you are V, even if you are overweight. Most structural abnormalities, like deviated nasal septum, scoliosis, bowlegs or knock-knees, are also due to Vata.

P people have medium frames with medium shoulders and hips, and normal joints. Their fingers and toes are medium in length. Their body frame and height are generally proportional and *balanced*, indicating a naturally prudent use of energy for development.

K people have a medium to broad frame with a *balanced*, bone structure and wide-set shoulders and/or hips. Their tendency to store energy encourages massiveness; football linemen are usually quite K in constitution. Their bodies seem well proportioned to the eye, with joints that are well lubricated and may be deep-set. Their fingers and toes tend to be short and squarish.

WEIGHT

Vata's *balanced*, promotes natural leanness of body. Some V people live out their lives in thinness and find it hard or impossible to gain weight, like my grandfather who could eat four meals a day and never gain an ounce. Such an individual's Vata expends all food energy that enters the body before it can be stored. V people are often skin and bones, with prominent tendons and veins on their limbs. Some Vs may overeat poor foods and become fat, but as they improve their habits and their diets and begin moderate exercise they can lose that weight and keep it off without much difficulty. V people are known for wide variations in weight even without radical changes in diet. They usually store most of their fat around their midriffs in a "spare tire."

Ps can usually maintain an average weight for their build, with minor fluctuations. They can usually gain and lose weight fairly easily, since Pitta is the body's principle of balance. They tend to deposit fat evenly all over their bodies.

K people can maintain moderate weight with regular exercise; otherwise Kapha's *balanced*, tends to make them add excess poundage. They gain weight easily, especially in the lower parts of the body such as the rear end and thighs, and lose weight with difficulty, since they innately enjoy having ample stored energy.

SKIN COLOR AND COMPLEXION

Your personal skin color depends greatly on your racial background. A Scandinavian who seems dark-skinned to his family will still be several shades lighter in pigment than the lightest black African. Compare yourself with members of your immediate family or with others who have the same racial mix as you do to make an accurate evaluation.

Vs tend to be naturally dark, or if lighter-skinned they tan deeply and do not burn easily. They usually adore heat and cannot get enough sun; they feel more "alive" after getting sun. Their bodies need regular infusions of heat thanks to Vata's *cold* nature, for Vata does not store enough energy to maintain good bodily warmth. Because of innately poor circulation V skin is usually cold to the touch and may have a grayish cast to it.

Ps have light-colored skin, often pink or coppery in hue. Because Pitta is *hot* and reactive their skin is usually warm to the touch. P circulation is strong but tends to elevated blood pressure. Ps freckle before they tan, and rarely tan very deeply. They do burn easily, and may suffer from sun allergy.

K people enjoy the sun and burn after overexposure, but adjust easily to intake of solar energy and tan evenly and thoroughly after moderate sunbathing. Their skin is cool but not cold to the touch, and because they have good circulatory tone they rarely suffer from cold hands and feet as Vs often do. They may have a few freckles, but never in P-profusion.

SKIN CHARACTERISTICS

Vs tend to have problems with *dry* skin because their elevated energy output quickly uses up any available external lubrication. Their skin may be dry all over, or dry in patches and oily in patches due to Vata's quality of *variability*. V skin chaps easily and may have a leathery texture to it. It is susceptible to conditions like psoriasis and dry eczema. Corns and calluses form readily, as do cracks, especially on the bottoms of the feet. V types often suffer from chapped lips. They may have a few moles or wrinkles. Their body hair is either scanty or overabundant, and tends to be dark, coarse, and curly.

Ps usually have delicate, *irritable* skin prone to rashes and pimples, and inflammations like impetigo. They usually have many moles, and their skin tends to wrinkle early. The body hair is light hued and fine-textured. Their skin is coppery-red in color, especially after exercise or when they are agitated. Their lips are deep red, reflecting the ample volume of blood beneath the skin. This also explains why Ps blush easily.

Ks have slightly oily, smooth, *thick* skin which is well lubricated, with a moderate amount of body hair and a mole or two. Ks are not naturally prone to any skin disorder. Their lips are full and moist.

SWEAT

V sweat is often scanty even in heat because the V body type is metabolically *cold* and has a natural need for external heat sources like stoves, steambaths and hot springs. V people who become overweight, however, perspire more.

Ps may sweat even in cold weather, because of Pitta's innately excessive *heat* production. Even P palms may seem sweaty.

K sweat is moderate, and is *consistent* even in climatic extremes.

HEAD HAIR

The hair and its luster are important indicators of overall tissue health, for healthy hair rarely grows on an unhealthy body. Hair is closely related to *Prana*, the body's vital force. This is the reason why, like Samson, none of India's rishis ever cut their hair. Instead they allowed it to grow as long as it liked and to break off whenever it chose to do so.

V hair is usually *dry*, but may *vary* from dry to oily in different spots on the head. It is ordinarily dark in shade and is coarse or rough in texture. V hair is usually very curly or even frizzy and tends to kink or tangle. It may be prone to dandruff or split ends and often seems dull and lusterless.

Everyone with naturally red hair has substantial Pitta in his or her prakriti. Other Ps are those people with light-colored (blonde or light brown) hair, or whose hair has gone grey or white at an early age. Early baldness is also a -P–indicator, since it indicates high levels of testosterone, a hot, aggressive, P–type hormone. P hair is usually thin and fine or delicate, and quite straight. Sometimes oiliness dims its luster.

K hair is most characteristically brown or dark brown or chocolatey and is thick and slightly wavy. It borders on coarseness. Oiliness is one of its chief disorders, but its luster is usually good.

NAILS

Vs have hard, brittle nails that are rough and may differ in size from one another. As always significant *irregularity* shows a significant degree of V. Their nails often display marked ridges or depressions and may be slightly bluish or grayish in color. People who bite their nails as a habit are often V types.

P nails are soft, strong, somewhat rubbery and well formed. Their color is a lustrous pink, with a coppery tinge due to the profuseness of *warm* blood right under the skin.

K nails are strong, large and symmetrical, in line with Ks natural *regularity* and lack of variation. They tend to thickness and may seem somewhat pale in color.

EYES

Your eye color is that wavelength of light the body does not desire and so reflects back instead of absorbing. Grey eyes, for example, indicate that the body does not need grey, and since grey is one of the colors associated with Vata, grey eyes in an organism suggest that it has ample Vata and needs no more.

Some people have brown patches in their eyes that indicate accumulated toxins in the system. These splotches do not represent the true eye color, though they may indicate a current condition. They should be ignored while determining constitution and only the underlying color considered.

Eye size is subjective. Everyone's eyeballs are roughly the same size, but the size of the head and the nature of the tissue that surrounds one set of eyeballs may make them seem larger or smaller than someone else's set. A K, like a deer, may seem to have large eyes, and like an elephant's the eyes of a V may seem small. Eyes that appear unusually close together or far apart are V in nature.

Grey, violet, and slate blue are the typical V eye colors. Very dark brown eyes, verging on the black of bittersweet chocolate, are also indicative of V. Individuals whose eyes differ in color from one another are usually V types. V eyes are often dry and scratchy. There is a grayish or bluish tinge to the sclera, and the eyes themselves quickly become dull and lusterless when the individual has expended all his or her energy and is out of sorts.

P eyes are medium in size and light in color. Hazel, green, red, light blue and those electric blue eyes that some red-haired persons have are all P eye colors. P eyes usually burn with an intense *fire* and radiate energy in all directions. The sclera is tinged reddish, and become fiery red when irritated.

K eyes are large and liquid, sometimes blue but more often milk chocolate in color. Their calm, cool, *stable* strength made the Ayurvedic texts compare them to the eyes of a deer or the petals of a lotus. They may have a tendency to itchiness.

MOUTH

V people tend to have crooked or uneven teeth, often with some teeth significantly larger than others. Buckteeth usually indicate Vata. Vata's *irregularity* may make the jaw too small to accommodate all the teeth, or too large for all the teeth to fit together snugly. V teeth tend to be brittle and over-sensitive to sensations like cold and sweets. V gums often recede early. The V tongue is often coated, and the coating is usually thin and adherent, and grayish or pinkish-grey in color. Vs may find an Astringent or Bitter Taste in their morning mouths.

P mouths have even teeth of medium size. Their teeth are prone to cavities, and their gums tend to bleed easily. Their tongues are coated occasionally, and the coating is usually yellow, orange or red. Sometimes the tongue is so *irritated* that it will bleed. The P mouth and tongue are also prone to canker sores. The early-morning P mouth may produce a Sour or metallic Taste.

Ks have large, even, gleaming teeth that rarely need attention. Healthy K tongues are rarely coated. When they are the coating is usually white, off-white, or greenish-white, thick and curdy, and associated with a sickly Sweetish or Sour-Sweetish Taste in the mouth.

APPETITE

V people are always anxious to eat, but their eyes are bigger than their stomachs; they feel full after eating less than they wanted to eat. Their appetites are *variable*: excessive hunger on one day may be followed by disinterest in food the next. People who become dizzy or faint unless they are assured of regular between-meal snacks are also Vs. They do not enjoy stringent fasting because their bodies do not store enough energy to carry them through long periods of food deprivation.

P people have good appetites and really enjoy eating. They are always ready to eat—morning, noon, night and midnight—and hate to miss meals. Ps become snippy or *irritable* if they fail to eat when they are hungry, for their systems are always on the prowl for new energy to consume and "manage." They are rarely fond of fasting.

K people have a *stable*, usually moderate desire for food, though they may be prone to emotional eating. They can go an entire day on water or juice alone without feeling any physical distress because they naturally store plenty of energy in anticipation of such periods of deprivation.

BREAKFAST

Vs often find it difficult to function efficiently if they miss breakfast, because by mid-morning they begin to feel anxious or sleepy as their blood sugar drops and their energy becomes exhausted. Many Vs notice that they burn up their food quickly and try to compensate with a heavy breakfast, but most feel better when they have a light breakfast and then an early lunch. Vs tend to rely on the caffeine in coffee or tea to wake them up and get them going in the morning. Unfortunately these insidious cups rob them of energy later in the day, and eventually exhaust them altogether by *drying out* their glands. V energy comes in spurts or bursts anyway, and artificial stimulation by caffeine or sugar exhausts the limited V energy reserves quickly.

P people can skip breakfast when necessary, especially if they are driving themselves toward some goal, but by lunchtime they begin to become hot and testy, and really calm down only after a good feed. Sometimes they suffer from heartburn when they are away from food for too long. They enjoy stimulants, and tend to misuse coffee and tea both in the morning to wake up and during the course of the day to maintain their high levels of energy expenditure.

K people find they do best with a light breakfast, like a piece of fruit, and often enjoy skipping breakfast entirely. They usually are not much perturbed even if they miss lunch. They are not naturally attracted to stimulants, but may enjoy a cup of coffee or tea in the morning to help mobilize themselves.

DIGESTION AND EVACUATION

For the purposes of this question anyone whose bowels do not regularly move at least once daily without straining or the use of laxatives can be considered to be constipated. A condition in which loose stools are passed three or more times a day constitutes diarrhea. Healthy bowels move once or twice daily without assistance.

Some V people are lifelong sufferers from constipation, with a tendency to hard, dark-colored stools and frequent gas or bloating. Other V types experience *variations* in their bowel habits, with periods of constipation alternating with spells of loose stools or diarrhea. Many V people know from experience that good eating habits are essential for good digestion. When they are constipated pure V people often respond only to strong laxatives like senna or castor oil.

P people are rarely constipated, and usually defecate regularly and frequently. Their stools are usually yellowish and well formed, but sometimes are loose and may seem *hot* and burning, especially after a hot, spicy meal. An intense yellow or orange stool indicates Pitta overload in the body. Many P people find that substances like milk, figs, raisins or dates act as laxatives for them.

K people are usually regular, and move their bowels once daily. They are sometimes slow in their elimination. Their stools are most often well formed but are rarely hard. When constipated they respond to medium-strength laxatives.

MENSTRUATION

V women tend to have very *irregular* cycles and may miss periods, especially if they exercise too much or their weight drops too low. The spacing between periods is often longer than a month. Their flow tends to be scanty, and there may be clots. Both these symptoms are due to Vata's *dryness*. The blood is usually dark in color. Constipation and severe cramps may develop just before the bleeding begins; sometimes constipation alternates with loose stools. The abdomen may feel tense and rigid. V cramps are generally more intense than are P or K cramps because cramping is itself due to Vata. Imbalanced Vata may create pre-menstrual anxiety, interrupted sleep, nervous tension, mood swings and "spaciness."

P women usually have regular cycles, but bleed for a longer time and more heavily than do others because of their innate *heat*. The periods may also be spaced closer together than four weeks. The blood, which may feel "hot," is usually an intense, bright red, but when Pitta is unbalanced it may show a bluish, yellowish or blackish tint. P women may have loose stools during or just before their periods, and may suffer from medium-strength cramps. Pre-menstrual Pitta imbalance may create irritability, intense food cravings, flare-ups of acne or skin rashes, headache (especially migraine).

K women often have effortless, regular periods with an average quantity of blood which may be rather light in color. K imbalance may add mucus to the blood. Any cramps are likely to be mild, and are dull rather than intense. K women tend to be prone to water retention. Premenstrual K imbalance promotes water retention, bloating, swollen breasts, vaginal itches, slow digestion and lethargy.

CLIMATE PREFERENCE

V-types are so *cold-blooded* that they love warmth at all times. It takes a lot of heat to make them sweat. The sun enlivens them, and they tend to lose strength during the dead of winter. Then they bundle up warmly and seek out external sources of heat to make up for their meager internal heat production.

Pure P people prefer the colder latitudes and find hot climates intolerable. Because they produce so much internal *heat* themselves they may love to sleep with the windows open even in winter. Mixed P types do not find heat so intolerable, but usually do prefer cold climates.

K types are *stable* enough not to be greatly disturbed by any extreme of climate, but if pressed often admit they prefer warm weather and are not overfond of high humidity.

SEX DRIVE

V types think a lot about sex, and sometimes find their fantasies so satisfying that they lose interest in physical consummation. When they do become interested they become intense. Their passion gets quickly inflamed and peaks quickly as they spend all available energy in the sex act. As with their other appetites their sexual appetite *varies* from day to day, though many Vs tend to fall into habits of sexual overindulgence which leave them exhausted. Their fertility tends to be lower than average.

P people, being *hot-blooded,* usually have ample sexual desire. They know what they want and when they want it, and readily put their desires into action. Whether their desire is great or small, however, Ps are able to balance their desire with its fulfillment. If their sexual gratification is thwarted or delayed their innate anger tends to flare up. Their fertility is average.

K individuals experience *steady* desire and normally enjoy sex without being particularly fascinated by it, for they are innately reluctant to "spend" energy. Once sex captures their attention, however, their appetites for sex intensify greatly. They are aroused to passion slowly but remain passionate for a long time once aroused. Their fertility is usually excellent.

PHYSICAL STRENGTH AND ENDURANCE

Though V types are so active that they are often restless, they tend to display low stamina. Vigorous exercise tires them quickly—it *dries* them out—and makes them feel hungry afterwards. Unfortunately they often drive themselves to excess and exhaustion through overactivity because they are convinced that "more is better," and because they love to expend energy when they have it. They may become addicted to vigorous exercise because it temporarily makes them feel calmly elated and pain-free. Their muscle tone is usually poor and they must give active attention to developing muscle coordination.

P people can endure vigorous exercise so long as it does not *overheat* them. Ps usually feel both hungry and thirsty after a good workout. When they want to they can pace themselves well, but being naturally compulsive and competitive they often refuse to recognize their limits. Their muscle tone and coordination are average.

K types have excellent muscle tone and are naturally coordinated. Of all constitutional types they are best able to endure vigorous exercise but many times they are least interested in it, reflecting their aversion to energy expenditure. Once motivated, though, they get great benefit from regular activity, and enjoy it because it makes them feel good. They rarely feel hungry after exercise.

PULSE

Pulse testing should be done early in the morning before eating. You should sit quietly with your back straight and your hands on your thighs for five to ten minutes before you test your pulse, breathing deeply and regularly so that the reading will be accurate. It is usually best to use your radial pulse, the pulse at your wrist below your thumb. Only three of your fingers are necessary for testing: your index, middle and ring fingers. Put your index finger closest to your thumb and your ring finger furthest away from your thumb, toward your elbow.

A V pulse is thin, shallow and *fast* with a broken or *variable* rhythm, or a tendency to skip an occasional beat. In purely V people this pulse seems to slither like a snake and the artery will feel hard and cool or cold to the touch. It is felt strongest under the index finger.

A P pulse is full, regular, and strong, with medium speed and rhythm; in purely P individuals it often seems to jump like a frog. The artery feels *warm* and soft. It is felt strongest under the middle finger.

The K pulse is strong, full, *slow* and rhythmic like the swimming of a swan, and the artery may feel cool and rubbery. It is felt strongest under the ring finger.

SLEEP

Usually light sleepers, V people may toss and turn and have trouble getting to sleep, or may wake up several times during the night for no apparent reason. Their ability to sleep *varies* greatly from night to night. Some nights, especially when they are exhausted, they will fall into such a deep, prolonged sleep that they are inert to the world and are almost impossible to arouse. Otherwise they tend to sleep fitfully and are easily disturbed by outside noises. Often, no matter how deep or prolonged their sleep, they wake up in the morning feeling unrested. Frequent sleepwalking or sleep talking is also indicative of Vata. People who grind their teeth at night are usually V types or are Vata provoked.

Ps go to sleep easily, sleep lightly and wake up alert. Even when they wake up during the night they can return to slumber quickly. Most nights they enjoy restful sleep, and can get by very well on a minimum of sleep for many nights in a row without seeming ill effect. When they do have trouble sleeping it is usually because of overattention to their work.

K types drop off to sleep quickly and sleep *heavily*, but wake up rested and alert. If permitted, they will gladly sleep many hours at a time; they save energy that way. Rarely does a K person have difficulty sleeping.

DREAMS

V types dream a lot and forget their dreams easily. In the morning they know they have dreamed but may only be able to remember fragments. Sometimes periods of seeming "dreamlessness" alternate with days or weeks of vivid dreaming. When they do remember, they often report violent, intense, active dreams, their minds continue to spend energy even when they should be resting. *Motion*, particularly flying in the air, is typical of V dreams, as is being pursued by something or someone.

P people can usually remember what they dream. Their dreams are often passionate or otherwise intense, and often involve heat, light or other energy. Usually the P individual is in control of the dream situation; if there is pursuit, it is usually the P person pursuing and not the other way round. Even dreams of buying and selling are P-type dreams, because they involve transfer of money ("green" energy). P people usually dream in color.

K people usually have very cool, calm, quiet, collected, uneventful, peaceful dreams, like those of an English countryside with cucumber sandwiches at afternoon tea in a gazebo on a swan lake. Ks usually do not bother to remember such dreams; they are more likely to recall those which are intensely emotional.

VOCAL QUALITIES

Untutored V people frequently speak in a breathy voice which becomes hoarse easily and cracks on strain. Voice training may overcome these natural defects. Vs tend to speak *quickly*, often with rising pitch at the end of a phrase, and tend to stray from the subject. They are usually very talkative and can speak on most any subject to most any audience, even if it is only the cat, the plants or a wall. They speak for the love of speaking. Talking expends a lot of energy, which is one reason they love it so. Their conversations may resemble monologues; in fact, two V people can spend hours talking at, not to, one another and both be satisfied afterwards without having communicated much. Part of their vocal weakness results from this overuse of their voices.

P people are usually concise and one-pointed in what they say. They know the message they want to deliver, the response they want to elicit, and the amount and type of energy they need to project to obtain that response. A P voice frequently carries in it a tone of impatience with the listener, and is usually intense; a P whisper can be clearly heard across a room. Two Ps are sure to communicate with one another when they meet, and they will often convert a conversation into a contest of wills to see who can outdebate whom. Ps are frequently accused of having *quickly*, tongues.

K types speak *slowly* and cautiously, without volunteering much. Information may have to be drawn out of them. A pure K will initiate a conversation only if he or she has something important to say, in contrast with the Vs who will strike up conversations with anyone and the Ps who will approach anyone who seems sufficiently interesting. K voices tend to be lower in pitch and intensity than the others but are usually more sonorous and melodious. Ks are a pleasure to listen to when you can get them to talk. Two Ks can easily sit across from one another for hours or days without anything more than a few perfunctory pleasantries passing between them. Perhaps their innate taciturnity helps preserve the sweetness of their voices.

CHARACTERISTIC EMOTION

This question concerns how you typically react when you are confronted by a stressful situation. You may not actually display this emotion if you have taught yourself not to, but your very first reaction is characteristic of your constitution.

Vs characteristically show *fear* or anxiety first, which is created by the *dryness* of their inherent Astringency. P types, full of the *heat* of Pungency, ignite into *anger* first, whether they show it outwardly or merely burn with it internally. K people like to avoid confrontations because of the *complacency* of their innate Sweet. They have a strong disinterest in change, and their emotional sensitivity often shows when stressed by unpredictable situations. Like ostriches, they hope that by ignoring a situation it will go away. It takes a lot to arouse them, but once aroused they may feel great fear or anger.

These proclivities tend to show themselves as first reactions to a situation in which some change in your environment is causing you to have to adapt. For an extreme example take the case of a friend of mine who one day walked carefree into a bank. One minute later a robber walked into the bank, pointed a gun at him, and said, "Hands up, you goof!"

In such a life-or-death situation a strongly V type would feel immediate fear and would put his or her hands up without delay. P types in this situation would raise their hands slowly in anger, thinking only of when they could have their revenge on the gunman.

My friend displayed the K response: he first experienced hurt at being called a goof, concluded that anyone who would call him a goof without knowing him was a offensive person, and decided to have nothing to do with such an insulting man. He therefore walked out the door of the bank, leaving the astonished bandit gaping behind him. A few yards down the sidewalk, as the emotion wore off, he realized that a robbery was in progress and called the police, who succeeded in nabbing the thief.

My friend's innate constitutional personality exerted a powerful effect on his behavior when he found himself having to adapt to dire straits. What effects must his prakriti be having on him, and our prakritis on all of us, during the less traumatic (and thus less noticeable) situations in which we all find ourselves daily?

PERSONALITY TRAITS

V types are sensitive, high-strung and react quickly to changes in their environments. They are exceptionally changeable, and resist regularity in their lives because their active minds demand continual stimulation. When their energy is high they can be the life of the party, but burn out quickly. Sometimes they crave companionship and other times demand solitude. They usually make friends easily, but their friendships are often short-lived. They love to travel for fun. Their hyperadaptibility gives them flexibility and a potential for detachment, but also tends to make them chaotic and "spacey." They find it difficult to concentrate on any one subject, and often fail to complete the projects they start.

V types recognize the need for self-development but are rarely consistent with any one program. They can become fanatic followers of cults or other far-out doctrines, but even their fanaticism is impermanent, and they may quickly and for little reason switch allegiance to a completely new set of ideas. Their faith often arises from insecurity.

P types are strong and forceful in their dealings. They are dedicated to the practical side of life. When permitted, they are domineering. They are inherently courageous and believe in fair play, and in a good mood exude exuberance, but when angry they can be cruel and hurtful. They make friends easily, especially if they perceive that such friends will be useful to them. They are usually acutely intelligent and tend to be *impatient* with anyone whose intelligence is not equally acute. Their innate arrogance of cleverness can make them intolerant.

P types are dedicated to their own self-development, which sometimes becomes a sort of ego-expansion. Their opinions are strongly held, and they can fall into fanaticism. They tend to stick with their fanatic ideas if they calculate that such a course would benefit them. Cult leaders and their lieutenants are usually P types.

Ks are predominantly calm, quiet, steady, serious sorts who most enjoy the pleasures of home and family. Patience, fortitude and humility are common K virtues. In excess these traits may engender passivity, attachment, possessiveness and greed. K people usually have very *stable* personalities, so stable that they sometime stabilize themselves right out of mental acuity or agility. They study each subject cautiously before committing themselves. Once committed to a course of action, though, they usually see it stubbornly through. They often make friends slowly, after deliberation, but a friendship established usually lasts.

Innate self-satisfaction makes K types less motivated for self-development than others may be. They do not make good fanatics, but their faith in whatever they believe is steady and unshakable, though it is often motivated by a desire to maintain the status quo. K types do tend to be innately more compassionate than others are, however. Perhaps they are more maternal because of the strong influence of the Earth Element in their characters. Mother Earth is Herself mainly Kapha in prakriti.

PREDOMINANT MODE OF PERCEPTION AND EXPRESSION

You can test your predominant sense by remembering your most recent vacation trip. Remember the experience; then ask yourself which aspect of the experience did you first remember. You may have taught yourself to organize your knowledge in a specific way, but your first reaction—your prakriti—usually reflects your constitution.

V people most often think predominantly in words. Even when they visualize (thinking in images) or emote (thinking in feelings) they usually use words to tie their thinking together. One reason for this is their acute sense of hearing, so acute that sometimes loud or dissonant noise can be physically painful to them. Vs usually are first struck by and preferentially remember sounds. A V who visited the coast might most easily recall seashore sounds, like the screeching of gulls or the rumble of waves.

P types are visually oriented, and visualize almost everything they think about.

They have no difficulty in creating fantasy images, for even if they have been trained to be verbal they will always try to see what they think about. Ps use images to relate words and emotions together, and tend primarily to remember images. A P by the sea might recall the whitecaps on the breakers or the glare of sunlight on sand.

Ks often think with their emotions and "feel" the connection between words and forms. Emotions often influence K thinking as much as or more than their physical "feel" for things. K people on the beach will find it easy to remember sensations like the sun's heat on their basking bodies or the water's wetness and motion against them as they swam. They are also likely to be able to correlate these tactile sensations with how they "felt" emotionally at the time.

THE MIND

Vs are good original theorists because they are not afraid to connect old thoughts in new ways. Their tendency to flit from idea to idea, however, makes it difficult for them to convert their theories in practicalities.

P people plan methodically and efficiently, and enjoy implementing new ideas dreamed up by more theoretical types. Ps love to engineer ideas into practical uses, and have little direct interest in the day-to-day details of running a project or business.

K types manage well. They are renowned neither for theorizing nor engineering, but give them an enterprise and they will make it run smoothly. If you have a factory or an office to run you will want a K in charge of it, unless that K's imbalance has translated into inflexibility or resistance to change.

MEMORY

Vs usually remember easily and forget easily. When angered they react just like a bottle of soda which is shaken and then opened: they erupt quickly, projecting all their energy into the anger, and as quickly return to normal when their attention is shifted from whatever it was that angered them. Within a short period of time they even forget why they were angry, unless whomever they blew up on reminds them.

Ps usually remember easily and forget with difficulty. A slighted P who explodes into rage will continue to smolder with indignation for a long, long time after the initial fire burns itself out. Ps often go so far as to manage their energy expenditure for the purpose of remaining angry longer.

Ks need to be told a thing more than once before it sinks in, but once they have learned it they know it for life. Like the elephant, they never forget. Also like the elephant it takes a good deal to irritate Ks, but once angered they never forget a slight.

LIFESTYLE

Vs find it difficult to create habits of any sort, even those associated with such naturally habitual behavior as eating and sleeping. Financial responsibility does not come naturally to them. Their innate diffuseness makes it easy for money to get spent as soon as it comes into their hands. They are prone to impulse spending on things they don't really need; they relate to money ("green" energy) as something to spend.

Ps plan and organize well, calculate their expenditures wisely, and spend sensibly. They are neither afraid to spend money nor to resist impulsive spending. They spend to further specific purposes, and tend to feel superior to those people who cannot exercise such self-control. Ps make or break all their habits according to their perception of a habit's utility to them.

Ks enjoy habits, sometimes to the extent of digging themselves into ruts. They always have money saved for that rainy day and can veer toward miserliness. They sometimes indulge in emotional spending, but usually feel that money is meant for accumulation.

Summaries of Constitutional Types

Count the number of V answers, P answers and K answers that you have obtained from this evaluation. Normally one or two of the Three Doshas will predominate clearly; these indicate your prakriti. For example, if you had 9 Vs, 13 Ps, and 3 Ks, your constitution is likely to be P predominant with V secondary. If there is confusion, consider especially your responses to these categories: body frame, skin color and complexion, head hair, appetite, digestion and evacuation, climate preference, dreams, characteristic emotion and lifestyle.

If you are still confused reflect on your preference for temperature. If you really hate cold and much prefer to be warm, your major predominance is very likely to be Vata. If you enjoy the cold because you truly cannot bear to be too hot, you probably have a Pitta predominance. If you are not naturally overtroubled by either, you are likely to have a substantial amount of Kapha in you, even if Pitta or Vata sometimes overshadows it. The summaries below may help you confirm your estimation of your own constitution:

VATA

V types are usually thin and have trouble gaining weight except when they overeat fanatically, which they may do to help stabilize themselves or to provide more energy for the next round of their activity. Their bodies are usually narrow in the shoulders and hips and their joints often make a cracking noise when they move them. They tend to be fidgety; fidgeting, like obesity, runs in families.

V people are dry. Their skin usually chaps easily and is prone to corns and calluses. Their hair tends to be coarse, dry and curly. V people suffer from cold, and often complain of poor circulation in their extremities. Their skin is usually cool or cold to the touch. They sweat little and love to be out in the sun.

Their appetites are irregular, and their love for excitement tends to lead them into irregular food habits that worsen their digestion. They usually suffer from or have suffered from chronic constipation, due to innate Astringency. They love soupy, oily, hot foods but always tend to go to extremes over their food, either overindulging in cheesy casseroles and heavy, hard-to-digest items, or denying themselves all heavy foods, or alternating between excess and denial.

They are prone to rapid fluctuations in their energy levels, their energy coming in spurts or bursts. Often they try to sustain this energy with Pungent stimulants like coffee rather than admit to themselves that they are tired and need to rest. Exhaustion inevitably follows periods of truly frenzied activity, but Vs may not recognize their fatigue until it forces them to rest.

V people often have difficulty with sleep. They may have trouble falling asleep or staying asleep, or they may evade insomnia by maintaining such a high level of exhaustion that whenever they do permit themselves some rest they sleep as if dead. Vs tend to feel pain more intensely than do other types, and loud noise is also less tolerable to them; their nervous systems seem to have less "insulation" than the norm. A Vs innate drive to avoid pain may manifest as fear. Vs adore oil massage because it helps soothe and quiet their overactive nervous system, which reduces their nervous sensitivity and therefore their pain, physical or mental.

V people live erratic lives because they find great difficulty in creating routine. The Bitter Taste makes them eternally interested in tinkering with themselves and their environment. If *changeability* characterizes most of what you do, you are V predominant.

PITTA

Pure Ps are Pungent, which makes them intense, hot and irritable. They are usually medium in height, weight and endurance. Their skin is usually light in color and reddens quickly in the sun, after exercise or when blushing. They sunburn easily and usually have plenty of freckles and moles. Their hair tends to be straight and light in color. Everyone whose hair is naturally red is at least partly P.

P people sweat easily because of all the heat they store inside. High inner levels of the Sour and Salty Tastes ensure that their appetites are always good. Fire's intensity gives them a love of food and confrontation; if they miss a meal they may "consume" some unwary bystander with their stored anger. They love all foods and usually digest food well. They have a tendency to loose stools and are rarely constipated.

Ps powerful fire makes the mind acute as well. P types tend to become quickly impatient around slower or less focused individuals. Ps usually sleep well because they feel it is sensible to do so, but if they become obsessed with work they may spend sleepless nights. They apply the same *intensity* and competitiveness to everything they do, in work or play, and the Pungent Taste makes them anger easily, even if they don't outwardly lose their tempers.

KAPHA

The typical K type is a heavyset individual who is a natural athlete when exercising properly and who gains weight just by looking at food when neglecting exercise. Most Ks remain healthy when they do enough exercise and do not overeat. The Sweet Taste being innately strong in their constitutions Ks really do not feel the intense physical hunger that Vs or Ps do, but they can become attached to food as a means of emotional fulfillment. K people sleep soundly and tend to oversleep.

K people generally do not crave the same excitement and stimulation that V and P people love, even from sex, although once they are stimulated the Sour and Salty Tastes become more predominant in them and their appetites awaken. K people are stable, somewhat slow, and tend to be complacent. Attachment to a stable, enjoyable status quo makes K people averse to change and may lead them to become greedy, stubborn or reactionary. Ks need motivation and stimulation just as Vs require balance and relaxation and Ps require a challenge.

DUAL CONSTITUTIONS
Individuals whose constitutions reflect the influence of only one dosha are really lucky in the sense that once they know themselves they can always know how they will react to specific stimuli. People with dual constitutions— VP, PK and VK—have personalities which are always in a sense "split": under certain conditions one dosha will predominate and under other circumstances the other dosha comes to the fore. The inherent cohesion of personality which characterizes purely V, P or K people is more difficult to come by for those of us who have dual personalities as we strive to balance the demands of two very dissimilar principles. Most individuals are dual in constitution.

VATA-PITTA
VP people generally have the poor circulation and love of heat that characterize Vs but their P nature sets definite limits to their ability to endure heat. The P in them makes them love to eat and the V ensures they will have trouble digesting large meals.

Many of a VP's characteristics show a combination of V and P; many of them have wavy hair, caused by a combination of Vs curliness and Ps straightness. Too often though the influences of V and P alternate in the VP individual. When a VP is unbalanced fear will often alternate with anger as a response to stress. This can lead to bullying and domineering. While the P aspect feels the need to command, the V presence creates self-doubt about the individual's capacity or fitness for command. Internal compromise may result in the domination of weaker beings.

A healthy, balanced VP weds the V capacity for original thought and the P expertise at application of theory. V and P have *lightness* and intensity as their common qualities. Proper direction of this intensity calls for harnessing the lightness for intensive self-development. Otherwise the V tendency toward addiction for pain control and the P predilection for addiction to amplified intensity will drag the VP individual into deeper states of addiction than either V or P people can separately know. VP types most need *stability*. They need to be weighted down with the heaviness that characterizes Kapha, the least influential factor in their personality equation. The Sweet Taste is most important for them.

PITTA-KAPHA

The PK constitution probably adjusts best to the confusion, irregularity and constant change that characterizes today's world. Many of the people who achieve all-round success in life are PKs who combine K stability with P adaptability. The active P metabolism balances the powerful K physique to promote good physical health, and the P anger is well tempered by K's cautiousness to encourage good mental balance. Though PKs usually prefer temperate climates they can easily endure extremes of heat or cold. They enjoy and profit by vigorous exercise, including sex.

The PK individual's dark side derives from the shared *oiliness* or wetness of P and K. The ease with which PKs succeed in the world promotes the arrogance and overconfidence of P and the smug self-satisfaction of K. These emotions can insulate the PK personality totally and efficiently from all realities other than the reality it wishes to perceive. Here the oiliness compounds the effect, for like "water off a duck's back" a PK may disregard criticism and acknowledge flattery alone. This attitude can make a successful PK very difficult to live with. Because Vata is minimized in them naturally PKs need the *dryness* of introspection or spiritual discipline and the irregularity of exposure to unpredictable situations to prevent overconfidence. Bitter and Astringent are their best Tastes.

VATA-KAPHA

Vata and Kapha are united in their *coldness*. Though they do not suffer as intensely from physical cold as do pure V types because of the strength and insulation of K they have a double emotional need for heat. They tend to be tall but reflect P norms in build and most other physical qualities. Their lack of heat usually manifests physically as digestive disturbances like constipation, and respiratory disease with much mucus production is also common.

VKs are usually zealous about what they do, and often overdo things by neglecting to use discretion. They can be by turns light, open and airy, and deep and secretive. Their diametrically opposite V and K natures and lack of a strong P fire make personality integration especially difficult for them. They must be especially wary of jumping to conclusions without proper preliminary investigation. The deeply emotional nature of K mated with the overactivated up-and-down nature of V ensures that emotional hurt goes deep and remains traumatic in a VK individual. VKs, who need *warmth* more than they need anything else, should employ more "hot" Tastes (Sour, Salty and Pungent) than "cold" Tastes (Sweet, Bitter and Astringent) in their diets.

PERCEPTION AND EVALUATION

Constitutions do not change, but perceptions may. After some time you may return to this evaluation and discover that your original opinion about your constitution was inaccurate. This is normal; as we become healthier our perceptions of reality become less distorted, and what may have seemed impenetrably incomprehensible before suddenly becomes profoundly pellucid. Use today's evaluation as the basis for planning your current health strategy. Even if you have erred today in determining your constitution you will find that living for a while according to your current condition is therapeutic.

The idea of constitutional types is simple, but not simplistic. Every individual has a body and mind that is quite unlike that of any other. Do not let these constitutional types bind you down into a stereotype. Take from them instead their perspective on some of your innate metabolic tendencies that are so deeply ingrained in you that they must be actively balanced if you are to remain in balance. Constitutional typing is meant to help you provide a foundation on which you can build the edifice of a new you. Vimalananda always said that if the foundation was good the structure would be good, and if the foundation was imperfect no amount of building could save the structure built on it. Constitutional analysis is the foundation of your road into personal enhancement.

Chapter Three
Food

Ayurveda teaches that food is the Prana, or life force, of living beings, and that life is a continual search for food. "Life lives off life," in the words of a Sanskrit proverb: we maintain our own lives by consuming other living beings.

In Nature's eyes all beings have an equal right to exist. If we wish to remain in harmony with Nature we should not carelessly slaughter Her other children. The taking of another's life, even that of a cauliflower, is an act which should be performed with sincere attention to its meaning. Sir Jagadis Chandra Bose, India's famous plant physiologist and physicist, proved more than fifty years ago that vegetables have sense organs that continue to function even after they leave the vine. The ancients agree that the carrot you crush for juice and the cabbage you chop to cook both feel pain and terror at being butchered and dismembered, just as any animal would. Plants cannot communicate their feelings to us, so we wrongly assume they have none. Vegetables and fruits have feelings too.

Few of us live our lives in a way that would make proud the turnip that was tormented for the table or the radish who relinquished its own identity to become an integral part of you or me. Eating is a sacred act, an offering made into the internal digestive fire in much the same way that offerings are made into external sacrificial fires. We make external offerings to propitiate cosmic forces personified into the forms of deities, and internal offerings to propitiate the indwelling spirit of a human form.

Each morsel of ingested food must give up its own individual existence and be transmuted so that it can participate in the greater existence of the human body. It is a mystery and a miracle: that which is "not-you" is converted by ahamkara into that which is part of you. Undigested food material that escapes into the body cavity causes an inflammatory reaction, but food material that is first digested and assimilated meekly undergoes adaptation into new body parts.

Any substance can act as food, medicine or poison for ahamkara. Food is that which nourishes the body, mind and spirit. Medicine improves the digestion to enhance nourishment. Poison impedes digestion and disturbs nutrition. Food is anything that you can dominate; medicine is anything that assists you in your domination; poison is anything that challenges this domination.

Some neurotics use food to provide them a sense of accomplishment, a macho sense of having successfully dominated, destroyed and assimilated another being. If in the outside world they are powerless, at the mercy of stronger beings who force them to act against their will, they are still the lords and masters of their private inner worlds and of all food-beings which enter therein. One reason that eating has been ritualized in India is to emphasize its sacramental aspect. Ritualizing eating helps limit this mental "bullying" by abasing the self-congratulatory personality in the presence of the Infinite.

Another reason for ritualizing mealtime is that each food article you eat alters your mental disposition. You are naturally attracted to those foods that create within you the state of mind that you desire, and naturally repulsed by those foods that produce opposing states of mind. Some foods, especially those derived from animal flesh, encourage your personality in its domineering and consumption. Beef and pork are the worst of all foods in this respect. Other foods, including especially milk, grains, raw fruits and vegetables, help to satisfy this unnatural craving and make you more willing to submit to the will of Nature. Your act of worship when you eat helps to minimize the negative qualities and enhance the positive attributes of your food.

The Ritual of Eating

Begin with your morning routine, paying particular attention to your urine, feces and tongue. Your urine should be clear and beer-colored and your feces light brown, with the consistency of a ripe banana. If your urine is turbid with a foul odor or your feces full of undigested food, offensive in odor and passed with abundant gas, ama is present. Any substantial coating on your tongue also indicates ama (toxins due to improperly digested food) in your digestive tract.

When such signs of ama, including nausea or heaviness of the limbs, appear you should fast for the day, or at least skip a meal. Never eat when you are not physically hungry. If you are not sure whether you have ever yet been physically hungry a day's fast will quickly teach you what hunger is.

Never eat when angry, depressed, bored or otherwise emotionally unstable, or immediately after any physical exertion.

Bathe, or at least wash your hands, face and feet, before you begin.

Sit while eating, in an isolated, clean, area. Face east if possible, the direction of the sun, the Earth's source of heat and fire. Eat alone, or with people you know and trust. Satisfy your sense organs by providing your dining room with pleasant music, fresh flowers, and the like.

Avoid habitual use of restaurants. Most people who sell you food are more concerned with their own profits than with your digestion. Satiation is not determined by how much you eat. A small amount of food presented to you lovingly will satisfy your soul, whereas large heaps of food from a fast-food restaurant may temporarily fill your belly but will leave your mind and spirit unsatisfied.

Only someone who loves you should be permitted to cook for you. Cooks in India are often selected from the priestly class so that there is at least some chance that while cooking some spiritually uplifting vibrations may be transferred into the food. Women should not cook when they are menstruating, which is a cleansing process; they should be relaxing instead.

It is best if your right nostril functions when you eat, since it increases your digestive fire. You can cause it to function by lying on your left side for a few minutes before the meal or by closing your left nostril with the middle finger of your right hand and breathing rhythmically through your right nostril for a few minutes. You can also change to your right nostril by plugging your left nostril or by hooking your left arm over the back of a chair.

Once all is in readiness, pray. Give thanks to Nature for providing you with food, and thank whichever deity you worship for being alive to eat it. Approach each food item with reverence and love, even if you are served something that you dislike but must eat. Suppose that you mother-in-law, whom you dislike, serves you rutabagas, which you hate. If wishing to maintain family peace you eat the rutabagas under duress those vegetables will carry your dislike and hatred deep into your system and disturb your balance. Consume your food, even if you dislike it, with respect for the sacrifice it is making for you, and it will carry the harmonizing power of your prayer inside you instead.

Before you begin your meal, feed someone else. Traditionally in India a five-fold offering is made: to the sacred fire, a cow, a crow, a dog and another human being, who might be a child, a beggar, or anyone else outside one's own family. This is a practical thanks to Nature, a feeding of some of Her children in gratitude to Her for providing you some of Her other children as sacrifices for consumption. And, it is another way of controlling ahamkara, an admission that the food is intended not for mere self-gratification but for the greater good of all beings. Feed anyone—a pet, a plant, a neighbor, a stranger—so you can experience a little of Nature's joy, the joy which a mother feels when she feeds her children and watches them grow and develop in consequence.

Immediately before you begin your meal chew some ginger to awaken your taste buds, start your juices flowing and purify your tongue and mouth. (P-provoked people should omit this step.) A good way to prepare the ginger is to slice it into long thin strips and marinate it in lemon juice with an optional pinch of rock salt.

Concentrate on your meal. No TV, radio, stereo or conversation should distract your attention. Observe silence while you eat; you can sit and chat afterwards.

Chew each morsel slowly and attentively many times. When feasible, eat with your hands so that your skin can send temperature and texture cues to your brain.

Feed all five senses by eating food that is attractive to the eye, tasty, aromatic, and pleasing in texture and sound (like the bubbling of a hot casserole or the hiss of a frying pancake).

After eating, drink a mixture of yogurt churned with water to support your digestive fire. People with weak digestion should use non-fat yogurt and a 1:3 proportion of yogurt to water; those with stronger digestion may use normal yogurt in a proportion of up to 3:1 yogurt to water. V people should add lemon juice and a pinch of salt and spice the mixture with fresh diced ginger or chilies, or whole or powdered cumin and coriander. P people should use coriander leaf or seed or cardamom powder, with less lemon juice and some sweetener like maple syrup or even sugar. K people should use honey with powdered ginger or black pepper, or other hot spices like diced green chilies. Anyone who is allergic to dairy products should omit this step, and some ancient authorities suggest that all dairy products should be avoided at a meal in which flesh is consumed.

At the end of the meal again give thanks, clean your mouth, apply water to your eyes to prevent weakening of vision because of increased Pitta at this time, urinate but do not encourage defecation, and then take a brief walk of 100 steps to promote digestion.

Avoid exercise or sex within an hour of food, and sleeping or studying within two hours. If you have overeaten, or if you are physically weak, lie for a few minutes without going to sleep on your left side to insure that your right nostril is working well to keep your digestion hot.

If at all possible, eat nothing after sunset. If you must eat at night, make it light. Eat no Kapha-producing food like melons, yogurt, sesame products, cheese or ice cream at night. Generally, all ice-cold food weakens digestion.

Your biggest meal of the day should ideally be at noon, when your digestive fire is strongest. Healthy Ks should eat one big meal and one smaller meal each day, allowing at least a six-hour gap between meals, and should not snack. Balanced Ps can if necessary schedule three meals daily, with gaps of four to six hours between them. They may snack if they retain a consistent four-hour gap. Vs should always eat small meals, three or four times a day, and may snack as needed with gaps of at least two hours. No one should allow less than two hours between any two meals or snacks because the gut requires at least this much time to ready itself for the next food deposit.

The Qualities of Food

All food is either *light* or *heavy* for digestion. Light foods include rice, mung beans, and wild meats like venison. Heavy foods include milk, black beans, raw fruits and vegetables, beef and pork. Cooking and preparation can alter these qualities; for example, milk becomes lighter when heated with saffron, and rice is made heavier by cooking with milk.

In general animal flesh is heavier than vegetables, legumes or grains; raw food is heavier than cooked; and preserved food is heavier than fresh. Raw food and cooked food should not be consumed together at the same meal, excepting small amounts of raw foods as appetizers or chutneys with a cooked meal, or small amounts of sauces or dressings on a raw meal. Do not mix heavy and light foods at the same meal; do not mix fresh food with leftovers. Very hot and very cold substances, like Mexican food and ice cream, should not be consumed together at the same meal.

Light food assists the mind's efforts to integrate body, mind and spirit because it pulls less blood down into the body during the digestive process. Heavy food requires more energy input to be digested; it draws more blood into the gut, leaving less for the brain to use. Rice is light, wheat is heavy. The wheat-eaters of North India are proud that they are more massively built than the rice-eaters of Southern India. The Southern Indians counter with accurate smugness that "wheat increases brawn, but rice increases brain." According to the Bhagavad Gita the food articles that most increase mental equilibrium when they are eaten in appropriate quantities and properly digested are rice, mung beans, milk, *ghee* (clarified butter), honey and pure water.

You may eat to your fill, but not beyond, of light food, but you must not eat more than one-half the quantity of any heavy food you might desire. People who are weak or ailing or sedentary or do not exercise should not take more than one-half their capacity of any solid food, no matter how light it is, and should take one-fourth their capacity as liquid. The remaining one-fourth of the stomach should be left empty to allow room for proper mixing of digestive juices with nutrients. Some authorities suggest that these proportions should be equal thirds.

V people are more likely to require cooked food than P people, who often do best on raw food. It is rare to find pure Vs who can balance themselves on a purely raw food diet, whereas many P or PK people can live almost indefinitely on raw food. VP people can usually exist comfortably on raw food during the spring and summer. Raw food helps tone up the digestive tract for K and VK people, but lack of intrinsic fire means that such people can overdo raw food.

V people do best of all on one-pot meals: soups, stews, casseroles and the like. In a stew, all the ingredients—meat, grain, legume, vegetable, fruit, spice— lose their own individuality and are welded into a single substance. Taken separately, each separate food demands different digestive attention from the body. Such foods may fight over this attention once they are inside the gut, causing indigestion.

Food combining is more important for V people than it is for other types. The V digestive system is not capable of handling a variety of foods at once, no matter how small the quantity, because the dryness and variability of Vata limits digestive responsiveness. Irregularity in diet disturbs Vata, and worsens digestion further. In a one-dish meal, however, the various foods have settled their differences in the pot, fought out whatever needed to be fought out, and come to some conclusion, which you then consume. One-pot meals are best for everyone during illness, convalescence and rejuvenation therapy.

Avoid all food articles which have been wrongly prepared, such as those which have honey baked into them, or which are overcooked, undercooked, burnt, unpleasant tasting, unripe, overripe, putrefied, stale and otherwise revolting. Deep fried food aggravates all Three Doshas. Vata increases because of the dryness developed during the frying process, Pitta increases because of the heat of the frying process and the rancid oiliness of the resulting food, and Kapha increases because of the heaviness of the oil and the stickiness of the food after frying. Deep fried food also impairs the eyesight, and should not be eaten regularly.

Every food you eat affects your mind as well as your body. The mind has three possible states:

Sattva, or *equilibrium*, the mind's normal state in which it discriminates accurately;

Rajas, or *motion*, a state in which excessive mental activity weakens discrimination; and

Tamas, or *inertia*, a state in which insufficient mental agility weakens discrimination.

Food which is putrid or vile in taste, or which is fermented, like alcohol, or has been preserved for too long, promotes Tamas. Legumes and other high-protein food like meat, fish and fowl increase Rajas, as do Pungent spices. Rajas and Tamas disturb mind-body-spirit integration. Sattva, which promotes this integration, is promoted by well-digested Sweet foods like grains and fruits, and by certain vegetables and dairy products.

Garlic and onions, which are both Rajasic and Tamasic, are forbidden to yogis because they root the consciousness more firmly in the body. Many people who follow a spiritual path also follow this restriction, which is fine so long as they remain healthy. When out of balance however they will often do well to use garlic, onions and other such substances to improve their body-consciousness, and return to strict spiritual food discipline when they have returned to health.

Eat food as directly from the farm as possible. Besides offering superior freshness and taste such produce has been through fewer hands to get to you. The food we buy in our cities has passed through the hands of the farmer, the dealer, the wholesaler and the retailer before reaching our tables. Each of these worthies has dealt with the food from a profit-making motive, not as a sacrament for sacrifice, and has thereby added negativity to the food. Negativity in food disturbs the mind.

Eating habits affect digestive capability. If for example you always eat cooked food, the day you eat raw food you will find it hard to digest because your system is not used to it. Some habits are good: the regular use of rice, wheat, barley, mung beans, daikon radish, ginger, onions, garlic, grapes, pomegranates, buttermilk or churned yogurt, ghee, rock salt and pure water is good for anyone whose constitution permits them. P people, for instance, should not make habitual use of garlic; it is too hot for them. Wild game is the only meat that is good for regular use.

Food articles to which you should *never* become habituated because they are too heavy to be properly digested include unchurned yogurt, pork, beef, mutton, dried meat, dried vegetables, molasses and cheese, as well as any foods which are very cold, very hot, thoroughly tasteless, or too intense in taste.

Meat is mandated in Ayurveda for debilitated patients, for warriors and for those who overexert themselves. But meat, which is very heavy for digestion, putrefies faster than other foods and produces ama quickly. Unless you exercise strenuously, regular meat eating will increase Fat rather than Flesh. It promotes speed rather than endurance, which is not good for Vata-affected individuals. Meat heats the mind and warms the body, but even in cold climates it ought not be used to excess. Most of today's meat is also of poor quality, taken from feedlot animals pumped full of antibiotics and other drugs who because they never exercised retained all their ama in their tissues.

Esoterically, the fear felt by the animal as it waits to be slaughtered and the hatred it feels for the human who slaughters it change the composition of its flesh and increase fear and anger in whoever eats it. The more the violence involved in the collection of our food, the greater the violence in our lives. Also, because digestive wastes are partly excreted in sweat, a meat-eater sits in his or her own body odor daily, breathing in chemicals which promote fear and anger, and projecting this fear and anger out at others. Not everyone can avoid meat, but when you can, you should.

Foods for Each Constitution

Every food substance has its own personality, a Taste personality, which inter-acts with and influences your consciousness. The knowledge of a food's Taste, Energy and Post-Digestive Effect makes it easier to predict its effects, which are complex enough not to be easily knowable in full. The food items listed below after each constitutional type are those items that are usually good for that constitution. The lists are not exclusive, and the observations made for each item are conditional on the eater's condition, including food allergies, digestive capacity and present degree of dosha aggravation. The nectar of immortality itself is poisonous to anyone who cannot digest it.

FOODS FOR VATA CONSTITUTIONS

Sweet, Sour and Salty foods are generally good for V people, since they sat-isfy the system and reduce its insecurity about being well fed. Bitter, Pungent and Astringent foods are less beneficial for Vata; they dry the system and inten-sify emotional instability, especially insecurity. Avoid large amounts of any Taste, for Vata is aggravated by excess.

Grains – Of all grains wheat is most satisfying to Vs, but it is heavy and easy to become allergic to. Well-cooked oats and rice are usually good. Buckwheat, corn, millet and rye all tend to be drying and so not as good for V as other grains, but because grain as a category is nourishing and therefore desirable for V people they can be consumed occasionally for variety. They especially must be cooked with plenty of water and with added butter, ghee or oil to reduce their dryness. Rice gruel is optimal for any whose digestion is catastrophic. Yeasted bread, filled as it is with gas bubbles after fermentation, is not a good staple food for V people. Unyeasted bread is better, but since bread of any sort is somewhat dried out by baking, freshly cooked grains are always preferable for V types.

Vegetables – The V gut prefers cooked to raw vegetables. Even some of the vegetables missing from the V list, like mushrooms, eggplant, peas and spinach, are suitable for V people if they are well-cooked and consumed only occa-sionally. Others that are found on the list, like onions and okra, often cause difficulties to the V person who consumes them raw. Most rough, hard vegetables like celery are better digested as juices. Salads of leafy greens like parsley, cilantro (coriander leaf, also known as Chinese parsley), lettuce, spinach and sprouts are all good for Vs on occasion if they are eaten with a good oily or creamy dressing.

Cucumbers, the squashes and zucchini can be consumed from time to time if they are cooked well with oil. Tomatoes are not good for Vs when raw, but tomato sauce cooked into a pasta meal, for example, may be suitable since the indigestible tomato skin and seeds have been removed. V types whose joints or muscles feel stiff and achey may be suffering from deep-seated ama, and should definitely avoid spinach, potatoes, tomatoes, eggplant and peppers.

Some of the best vegetables for V types are:

Asparagus, Beets, Carrots, Celery, Garlic, Green Beans, Okra, Onion, Parsnips, Radishes, Rutabagas, Turnips, Sweet Potatoes, Water Chestnuts

Fruits – Most fruits are good for Vs, except those that are naturally Astringent like cranberries and pomegranates, or those that are drying, like apples. Cranberry sauce and pomegranate syrup are however acceptable, as are stewed or baked apples or applesauce. Sweet pomegranate juice is permissible. All dried fruits, even the Sweet ones like figs and grapes, are inappropriate for Vs unless they are reconstituted to normal juiciness by soaking in water, or better yet by stewing, which heats them up as well.

Unripe fruits should be avoided, especially bananas, which are Astringent when unripe. Ripe bananas are good, however, because judiciously used they can control either diarrhea or constipation and are soothing to the gut. Mangoes and apricots are especially good. Overuse of melons may cause disturbance of both Vata and Kapha, and can be prevented by eating fennel, clove, black pepper or red pepper on the melon as an antidote.

Good fruits for Vs include:

Apricots, Avocados, Bananas, Berries, Cherries, Coconut, Dates, Figs, Grapefruit, Grapes, Lemons, Mangoes, Melons, Nectarines, Oranges, Papaya, Peaches, Pears, Persimmons, Pineapples, Plums

Flesh Foods – Vs are the only people who truly need animal foods in their diet. They need the complete proteins these animal foods provide. Overindulgence in animal flesh, though, quickly weakens the sensitive V digestion. Even if it is well digested, long-term use of any high-protein food always increases Vata, since the residues of protein digestion add to the body's nitrogenous waste burden.

Many Vs are able to fill their need for animal protein by judicious use of dairy products. Otherwise eggs, chicken, turkey, fresh fish and venison are all generally good for Vs. The only commercially available red meat they should eat is goat or lamb, which sometimes can help provide temporary balance to the system. Goat is good for V people; lamb should not be consumed regularly.

Beef is permissible when absolutely necessary to "ground" the V person imme-diately. Care should be taken with shellfish because of its potential to cause allergies. Eggs should be scrambled, with milk if possible, or poached; fried eggs are not fit for regular consumption.

Legumes – Legumes are the vegetable kingdom's equivalent of meat. They are high in difficult-to-digest protein, whose metabolic by-product is nitroge-nous waste. Nitrogen is a gas, and all gases increase Vata. Nitrogen has even been shown to be essential to the development of certain cancers that hate oxygen. High-protein wastes are doubly dangerous in that they also leach cal-cium from the system as they are expelled, thereby potentially weakening the bones. To prevent these undesirable results it is best for everyone to avoid overindulgence in any kind of protein. Mung beans are the best of all high-protein foods because they are the lightest for digestion and disturb the mind least. Peanuts encourage the blood to clot and should not be eaten by any-one whose circulation is already impaired.

Cook legumes with turmeric to prevent them from polluting the blood; with cumin and coriander seeds to enkindle the digestive fire; and with ginger, gar-lic or asafetida to prevent Vata from being disturbed. Add a little oil to the cook-ing pot for this same Vata-controlling purpose. Increased Vata due to beans and peas usually comes in the form of intestinal gas, which can be reduced by soak-ing the legume for at least an hour and throwing out the soak water before cooking. If they are still too gas-producing boil them five to ten minutes in an excess of water and discard that liquid also before starting to cook them.

In India, peas and lentils are most often used split. Splitting exposes more surface of the legume to the cooking process and eliminates the indigestible outer coat. The best way to use these split pulses is to cook them into a well-spiced soup and consume them with grains. If you cannot locate split peas and beans you can sprout them first and then wash off the hulls.

Vs should eat only a small amount of legume at any one meal. Even tofu, which is pre-digested, can aggravate Vata if consumed daily in large amounts over a long period of time. The best legumes for V people are black lentils, red lentils, chickpeas, mung beans and tofu. Black lentils are very strengthening but are also very heavy to digest. They must be well soaked before cooking and must be cooked with extra garlic or asafetida.

Nuts and Seeds – Almonds are the best of all nuts. They should never be eaten with their skins, which irritate the lining of the gut, nor should they be blanched in hot water. Soak them in lukewarm water overnight and peel them the next morning. Some claim that ten almonds each morning provide the body with enough nutrients for the whole day. Pumpkinseeds are a brain tonic. Being heavy for digestion, overuse of sesame products gradually ruins the tone of the gastrointestinal tract. All nuts and seeds are good for V peo-ple, but are too concentrated for regular use unless they are made into nut and seed butters or milks. Food that is too concentrated resists penetration by digestive juices and is one of the chief causes of Vata-caused indigestion.

Oils – In general, sesame is the best oil and safflower oil the worst, but all oils are good for V. Almond oil is good for the brain, coconut and sesame oils for the hair, and mustard oil for the skin.

Dairy – All dairy products are good for V types who are not allergic to them. Hard cheeses should be eaten sparingly; because they are so compact and concentrated they should be cooked into a more liquid form, like fondue or chile con queso. Yogurt blended with water and spiced with ginger, cumin or the like helps remove Vata from the system.

Sweeteners – Sweet reduces Vata. Vs can use any sweetener in moderation except white sugar, which is poisonous for them. Honey may be used freely but must never be cooked. Overuse of Sweet eventually increases Vata.

Spices – All spices, and especially ginger and garlic, are good for Vs and VKs in small quantities. Vs are always tempted to overuse spices, hoping to improve their digestive capacities, but overuse of hot spices eventually aggravates Vata. VP people should be cautious of spices; the V aspect of their natures craves them but they can seriously aggravate the P aspect. Asafetida is one of the best spices for Vata control, but should not be used by anyone whose liver or mind are too "hot." Cold fennel or sandalwood tea can overcome the ill effects of asafetida in a V person; pomegranate and apple can be used for the other dosha types.

Vices – This category is included because human beings do fall prey to vice now and again. If you are going to sin you should at least do so wisely, and avoid falling prey to guilt or side-effects. No one should ever use any intoxicating substance habitually.

V people are prone to addiction. They should avoid all vices, including especially tobacco, sugar and caffeine. Half a glass of wine diluted with water, with or after a meal, is beneficial for a V person; larger quantities of alcohol can be deadly. Vs should avoid all wines that they know contain chemical additives. Beer is not as good as wine for Vs because of its yeast content, and hard liquor is too intense for the V constitution. Intensity is itself intoxicating to V people, but intensity encourages inconsistency. Relaxation and meditation are better.

FOODS FOR PITTA CONSTITUTIONS

P people should avoid Sour, Salty and Pungent, the "hot" Tastes, and should concentrate on Sweet, Bitter and Astringent, the "cold" Tastes. If Vs should especially avoid caffeine and sugar, Ps should especially avoid meat, eggs, alcohol and salt. All these substances augment Pitta's natural aggressive and compulsive tendencies. Grains, fruit and vegetables cool the Pitta heat and should form the majority of the P diet. Vegetarianism is best for P people; every pure P should make a sincere effort to become vegetarian.

Grains – Barley is the supreme grain for P people because it is both cooling and drying, and helps reduce excess stomach acid. Rice comes next, followed by oats and wheat. Buckwheat, corn, millet and rye are all heating and should not be consumed habitually by Ps. Yeasted bread is not good for Pitta because of the sourness produced during fermentation, but unyeasted breads are good.

Vegetables – Ps can eat vegetables all day long, and should concern themselves only to avoid Sour vegetables like tomatoes and Pungent vegetables like radishes. Tomatoes in all forms are forbidden. Garlic should be avoided. Beets, carrots and the long white radishes called daikon purify the liver and help Ps control Pitta as long as Pitta is not already increased. If Pitta is disturbed they should be avoided.

Steamed white or yellow onions are good on occasion for P people because these onions even though they are Hot, lose their Pungency on cooking and become wholly Sweet. Red or purple onions are too Pungent for Ps, as are all varieties of peppers. Creamed spinach or spinach with cottage cheese is usually satisfactory for P types. Even normally permitted vegetables like parsley should be avoided if for reasons of age or growing conditions they taste unusually Sour or Pungent. Likewise, even vegetables that are not listed below are permissible when a particular specimen is unusually Sweet.

Ps do best with these vegetables:

Asparagus, Broccoli, Brussels Sprouts, Cabbage, Cilantro, Cucumber, Cauliflower, Celery, Cress, Green Beans, Leafy Greens, Lettuce, Mushrooms, Okra, Peas, Parsley, Potatoes, Sprouts, Squashes, Water Chestnuts, Zucchini

Fruits – Ps should eat Sweet fruits and avoid Sour fruits. Any piece of fruit on the list below which might happen to be Sour should not be eaten; this especially includes apples, cherries, grapes, oranges, pineapples and pomegranates. Likewise, any fruit like berries that are not on this list may be eaten if they are exceptionally Sweet. Papaya is generally too "hot" for the P constitution. Bananas, even though they are Sweet and reportedly help cure ulcers, have a Sour Post-Digestive Effect and should not be eaten regularly by P types. Figs and grapes are especially good for Ps, since they both are Sweet and act as laxatives. The grape is the Queen of Fruit, and the mango the King. Even though lemons and limes are Sour they reduce Pitta if used sparingly; overuse, especially of lemons, will however increase Pitta.

The following fruits are best for Ps:

Apples, Apricots, Avocados, Cherries, Coconut, Dried Fruits, Figs, Grapes, Lemons, Mangoes, Melons, Nectarines, Oranges, Peaches, Pears, Persimmons, Pineapples, Plums, Pomegranates

Flesh Foods – P people should avoid all seafood, which is "hot" and tends to cause allergies. Egg yolks are hot, and egg whites cooling. Ps can digest flesh foods but should generally avoid them since they pollute the blood and encourage aggression and irritability. Chicken, turkey, rabbit and venison are permissible for P people.

Legumes – While P people digest most foods well they should be wary of legume overconsumption because the same nitrogenous wastes which aggravate Vata also aggravate Pitta with their acidity. However, in small amounts all legumes except red and yellow lentils are good for them. The best legumes for Ps are black lentils, chickpeas, mung beans and tofu.

Nuts and Seeds – Most nuts and seeds are too hot and oily for P types. Coconut is good for P people because even though it is oily it is also very cooling. Freshly squeezed coconut milk is excellent for aggravated Pitta. Sunflower seeds and pumpkinseeds are also permissible.

Oils – Ps may consume small amounts of almond or flax oil, and larger amounts of coconut, olive or sunflower oils, but should avoid oil excess.

Dairy – All Sweet dairy products, like milk, unsalted butter and ghee, are good for P types; no Sour products are. Yogurt can be consumed if it is spiced with cinnamon or with coriander and a few drops of lemon juice, a sweetener is added, and it is blended with equal parts of water. P people should use soft, unsalted cheeses; hard cheeses should be strictly limited.

Sweeteners – Pitta is relieved by sweets. Of all people Ps can best handle Sweet food, including sugar, because sweets reduce heat. This is why residents of hot countries can eat more sugar and suffer less for it than can residents of colder climes. Molasses is "hot" and Ps should not use it. Long-term overuse of honey, which is also "hot," could theoretically aggravate Pitta.

Spices – Spices increase the typical P aggressive impatience. Ps should resist the temptation to become addicted to hot spices and should use only the cooling spices listed here. Mustard should be eliminated, and salt eliminated or drastically reduced, from the P diet. Cumin, being hot, is always used with coriander for balance. The best spices for regular use by P people are cardamom, cinnamon, coriander, fennel, and turmeric and small amounts of cumin and black pepper.

Vices – Tobacco is too hot for the P system, as is alcohol. An occasional beer may, however, help a P relax. Black tea is Astringent and may be used occasionally. Coffee is Pungent and irritating to the liver, and must not be used habitually. Prolonged use of coffee weakens the digestive fire and overheats the blood, producing such symptoms as emaciation, headache, palpitations and breathing difficulty. Treatment for coffee addiction must address both Vata and Pitta, and should employ milk, ghee and butter freely to antidote its effects.

FOODS FOR KAPHA CONSTITUTIONS

K people need to concentrate on Bitter, Pungent and Astringent foods which invigorate their bodies and minds, and should avoid Sweet, Sour and Salty substances which help them remain set in their ways. Ks should never eat fried or otherwise greasy food, and should shun dairy products. Fat is the worst possible food for K types. Vegetables are best for balanced Ks, who should limit the total amount of food they eat.

Grains – K people need grain less than do V or P people. The hot, drying grains buckwheat and millet are best for Ks, followed by barley, rice and corn. K people do best with roasted or otherwise dry-cooked grains. All breads should be toasted, or better yet avoided. Wheat is too heavy, cold and oily to be good for Ks.

Vegetables – All vegetables are good for K except potatoes, tomatoes and water chestnuts. Cucumbers, though Sweet, are also Bitter and Astringent and therefore do not aggravate Kapha. K people should avoid very Sweet, very Sour, and very juicy vegetables. Otherwise they can eat as many vegetables as they like as often as they like. Leafy greens and vegetables which contain seeds (like squashes) should get preference over root vegetables, which are naturally more Earthy. Raw vegetables are good; steamed or stir-fried vegetables are easier to digest. Peppers are good for K types. K people who overdose on chilies, cayenne, or other hot Pungent spices may use ghee to antidote any resulting Pitta aggravation.

Fruits – K people should avoid both very Sweet and very Sour fruits, and any fruits which are very juicy. Dried fruits like prunes are good. The best fruits for Ks are apples, apricots, cranberries, mangoes, peaches, pears and pomegranates.

Flesh Foods – K people rarely need any flesh foods because their flesh is adequately nourished by other foods. When they do eat flesh it should be roasted, broiled, baked, or otherwise cooked dry, but never fried. They may eat chicken, eggs, rabbit, seafood and venison.

Legumes – K people should not overeat legumes any more than they should overeat meat; their bodies do not require large quantities of protein. Legumes are much better for Ks than meat, though, because of the lack of animal fat. K people should however avoid the heaviest of the legumes, such as black lentils, kidney beans and soybeans. Well-cooked tofu is permissible for Ks in small quantities, since larger quantities are likely to increase Kapha. The best legumes for K people are black beans, mung beans, pinto beans and red lentils.

Nuts and Seeds – K people do not need the heavy, oily energy of nuts and seeds and should avoid them. They may eat sunflower seeds and pumpkin-seeds on occasion.

Oils – K people should avoid the use of oils. They may use almond, corn, safflower or sunflower oils when necessary.

Dairy – K types do not need the heavy, oily, sticky, cooling qualities of dairy products, which are very like Kapha's own qualities. Small amounts of ghee are good. Goat's milk is better than cow's milk because it is "hotter." Goat's milk is lighter for digestion than is cow's milk, and does not promote respiratory disease as cow's milk sometimes can.

Sweeteners – Kapha is increased by sweets, and Ks should not use any sweeteners except raw honey, which helps reduce Kapha.

Spices – Ks find spices useful to awaken their organisms; they can use all spices except salt, which increases Kapha directly. As for V people, ginger and garlic are best for Ks.

Vices – Only pure K people can really benefit from occasional use of stimulants. Black tea is good for them, and coffee is acceptable. Occasional smoking is not as bad for Ks as it is for Vs or Ps because the heat and subtlety of the smoke can help reduce Kapha. Overindulgence in smoking is certain to increase Kapha, however. K people really do not need to use alcohol at all. When they do they should avoid beer and drink only wine or diluted hard liquor. Only pure Ks should touch hard liquor.

The above suggestions are guidelines only. You will have to discover for yourself which rules are most important for you to follow and which can be ignored safely on occasion. As far as possible you should avoid the foods that are inappropriate for your prakriti, but when you want to cheat you should cheat at the right time.

P people who want to eat hot spicy food should not do so at noon or in the summer, when Pitta is at its height, but only in the early morning or the early evening during the fall or winter when Kapha can cover for them. K types who want to enjoy heavy, sticky food should avoid morning and evening, winter and spring, and eat it only at noon in the summer when Pitta can help them digest it. Vs should not eat Vata-promoting junk food in the afternoons or in autumn when Vata naturally predominates; they should stick to morning or noon in spring or summer, when the influence of Kapha or Pitta is greater.

DUAL PRAKRITIS

Generally a VP person should follow a Vata-controlling diet in fall and winter and a Pitta-controlling diet in spring and summer. Since Pungent increases both Vata and Pitta and Sweet controls both these doshas, VPs should especially avoid spicy, Pungent food and the anger they create, and search instead for Sweetness in everything they do and consume.

PK people should follow a Pitta-controlling diet from late spring through early fall and a Kapha-controlling diet from late fall through early spring. Bitter and Astringent and their associated willingness to accept change and lack of security are best for PKs, because both Tastes control both Pitta and Kapha. Sour and Salty and their envy and hedonism are doubly dangerous for PK people because both increase both Pitta and Kapha.

VKs should concentrate on controlling Vata in summer and fall and controlling Kapha in winter and spring. Since both Vata and Kapha are cold and need heat, VKs should prefer Sour, Salty and Pungent, the "hot" Tastes, to Sweet, Bitter and Astringent, the "cold" Tastes. In summer and fall Sour and Salty may be preferred but should be balanced with Sweet. In winter and spring Pungent may be preferred but should be balanced with Bitter and Astringent.

Specific Food Items

Brown rice is full of nutrients, true, but polished rice has been preferred in India since time immemorial. Brown rice is too rough in texture for most V people, too hot for many P people, and too heavy for the average K person to use regularly. In most parts of India where rice is the staple grain it is parboiled before it is polished. This parboiling drives the vitamins and minerals deep into the grain so that only small amounts are lost during the milling process. If you choose to use polished rice ensure that it was parboiled before polishing.

Milk is meant for people who have strong digestion fire and who are either very sexually active or who are emaciated from some other Vata-producing activity and need rest and sleep. Mung bean soup can be used as a substitute if milk is unavailable or inadvisable. Some yogis live on milk alone because it is the only food given willingly through joy by any being for the purpose of nourishing another. Fruit and honey, which are also foods that are meant for other beings, are not relinquished willingly, and their use by humans may deny their original recipients a chance at life. All other foods, including nuts, seeds and grains, involve the killing of another being.

Milk improves its drinker's mind by encouraging motherliness, and helps integrate the body's consciousness with that of the mind and spirit. Plant protein is so different in composition from animal protein that it is sometimes insufficient to ground the consciousness firmly in the physical body. Other animal protein, derived from flesh, drags the consciousness down into the flesh, which discourages it from that breaking free of earthly restraints that is required for spiritual advancement. Milk is the one food that combines the Sattvic essence of plants with the firm groundedness of animals.

Some authors argue that milk is useful only for young animals and should not be consumed by adults. It is true that some people are genetically incapable of digesting milk properly, and that others develop milk intolerances as they grow. But milk is not bad for every adult. Dairy products are important to the diets of most Central Asian nomads, and the traditional menu of the Masai tribe of Kenya is perhaps 95% milk. Masais, though dreaded as warriors, never kill the animals of the jungle, and only rarely slaughter their cattle for food. Is it possible that centuries of milk consumption have encouraged them in this attitude that all beings have a right to live?

Milk is wrongly blamed for the many ills that can arise when it is improperly consumed. Milk should not be:

Drunk cold. Milk is Cold in Energy, and serving it at refrigerator temperatures compounds its coldness and heaviness.

Homogenized. Homogenization changes the fat and makes it almost indigestible, which encourages ama formation.

Consumed with other food. Milk is a complex, complete food and should be taken alone, or with ghee and honey. It may however be cooked with certain other foods like grains.

Overconsumed. You should not ordinarily expect your system to deal well with more then 12 oz. (33 cl) of milk at a time.

Unspiced. Turmeric, ginger, cardamom, cinnamon, nutmeg, clove and saffron all improve milk's digestibility, especially in the presence of honey, which reduces milk's Kapha-producing tendency.

Honey is both medicine and food. Like poison it spreads immediately throughout the whole body, penetrating to the deepest tissues without having to be first digested. Poison ruins the body's tissues, however; honey, being predigested to act as food for baby bees, nourishes the tissues. Honey is good for the heart and the eyes, promotes healing of the wounds to which it is applied, removes poisons from the body, and transports herbs added to it deep into the tissues. It is also aphrodisiac. Honey should *never* be used in cooking or baking, as extreme heat increases its poisonous qualities and makes it produce ama in the body. It is better to bake with barley malt, rice bran syrup or date sugar.

Ghee and honey potentiate each other when taken together, but they should never be mixed in equal quantities. Take more ghee than honey (at least 2:1) if you want improved tissue nutrition, and more honey than ghee (at least 2:1) if increased digestive capacity is your goal.

Butter is tonic to the brain, especially after it has been clarified into ghee. One tablespoon of melted ghee with half a teaspoon of sugar or maple syrup early in the morning helps promote mental coolness in P types. Replacing the sugar with a teaspoon of honey helps promote mental cohesion in V types. Ghee increases the digestive fire without increasing Pitta, helps to remove the effects of poisons, promotes beauty, improves the complexion and luster, and is aphrodisiac. It promotes mental stability and intelligence and is a good vehicle for most herbs.

Salt is intense, hot, heavy and oily. Used in excess it ages the body quickly, promoting wrinkles, baldness and patchy falling of hair, producing diseases of blood and flesh, loosening the muscles and joints, and promoting weakness, lethargy, debilitation and a decreased capacity to work. Reducing salt in your diet can make you live longer and healthier. P and K people especially should try to eliminate salt from their diets, and Vs should eat just enough salt to keep their digestive fires hot. The best of all salts is *saindhava,* a variety of rock salt from the Sindh region of Pakistan. Saindhava is said not to cause the body to retain water as most salt does.

Yogurt increases Kapha because its qualities are almost exactly the same as those of Kapha. Honey reduces yogurt's Kapha-forming qualities, and spices antidote it even further. The addition of water to this spiced yogurt dilutes it, and churning breaks up its gel structure to make it less slimy and viscid. The resultant mixture aggravates Kapha very little and promotes digestion greatly. Everyone who is not allergic to dairy products should drink a cup of it at the end of each meal.

Addiction and Taste

Humans frequently become habituated to foods that do not agree with them but do intoxicate them. A V person's love of sugar, which provides instant satisfaction and temporarily controls the mental eccentricities that Vata creates, may make that V person hypoglycemic. P people may become habituated to meat or to hot spices that inflame Pitta and make them more obsessive, intense, goal-oriented and driven. K people may habituate themselves to heavy, fatty foods that reinforce their natural complacency.

All of us use our food to affect our consciousness; most of us, though, prefer to perpetuate all our old idiosyncrasies and personality traits instead of improving them with a diet balanced according to individual constitution. We live in a fast world in which many of us try to run even faster than the world forces us to. Once an individual has invested so much in his personality that he feels he can no longer afford to change it he will search for crutches to help maintain his pace. Whenever you use a crutch, though, you run the risk of becoming dependent upon it.

We can become addicted to almost anything. Though substances differ in their power to addict, all our addictions are fundamentally identical. We addict ourselves to thrills, and it appears that all thrills are mediated by similar chemical changes in the brain. Inspiring music, works of art, Nature's glories, films, ballets, plays, books, sports events, parades, perfumes, food, gambling, exercise, sex and everything else which overwhelms you with tingling excitement give you pleasure because of internal molecules.

Some researchers believe that thrills occur when molecules called endorphins are released. A drug called naloxone blocks those molecules and prevents music from inspiring you, movies from stirring you, and parades from creating a lump in your throat. Other researchers credit adrenaline, dopamine and other hormones with thrills, and some like Vimalananda regarded increased blood flow into certain sections of the brain as the cause of exaltation. Whatever the specific cause, chemistry is at the basis of all our thrills and addictions.

Our society is inundated by addictions because we crave intensity and require ever-stronger thrills to satisfy our cravings. Humans who become addicted to intensity can exhaust their internal thrill molecules, and then may turn to certain foods for stimulation, or may use drugs as substitutes. Addiction to drugs reduces sensitivity to the simpler thrills of life, and weakens our very humanity. Female rats administered morphine lose all maternal instinct and refrain from showing maternal behavior to their offspring. Naloxone returns their behavior to normal. Endorphins, which are internally derived opiates, may have a similar effect to morphine. We cannot afford to purchase painlessness at the cost of maternal instinct; we are dependent for health on Nature, the Universal Mother.

Subtlety has gone out of fashion in our society. Our nervous systems are no longer sensitive enough to function at the level of "art, grace and culture" which for Vimalananda distinguishes human beings from animals in human form, those who have lost interest in differentiating between right and wrong.

Animals also self-administer drugs to themselves on occasion. Baboons have been known to use tobacco; elephants, raccoons, bears, goats, pigs and sheep consume fermented fruits and grains for the alcohol; and reindeer, cattle and rabbits sometimes partake of intoxicating mushrooms. Animals in the wild know when to stop, though, for they use their intoxicants only for an occasional change of pace. Many humans do the same, but others train themselves to live at their drug's pace. Like those lab mice who become so addicted to cocaine that they will prefer the drug even to food and water, humans rarely stop willingly once they have dedicated themselves to intensity.

Any habit that you cannot break without seriously damaging your body, mind or spirit persona is an addiction. V people usually become addicted to substances that reduce their pain and insecurity. P people adopt addictions that keep them at the high level of activity that they associate with success. K people often fall into addiction unawares because of poor eating habits that they fail to change.

SUGAR

All addictions are fundamentally addictions to the Sweet Taste, the Taste that creates satisfaction in ahamkara. Each addiction develops under individual conditions and requires individual consideration for its removal. All addictions must be broken, though it is usually best to break them gradually so that neither ahamkara nor its organism will go dramatically out of balance in the process.

Addiction to sugar is a good example of how addictions develop. If you search for satisfaction primarily in your food instead of in your life you may well become addicted to sweets. If you are not careful to select healthful Sweet foods like fruit and whole grains, you will probably fall prey to sugar-filled junk foods like doughnuts for your Sweet fix. When you eat too much white sugar for too long it will exhaust your system's ability to digest it. This will make you hypersensitive to it, which will aggravate Vata. Vata, which increases with any sort of exhaustion and hypersensitivity, will then exaggerate the gap between your high blood sugar level and your low blood sugar level. The size of this gap will depend on the intensity of your Vata disturbance and will determine in turn the severity of your symptoms. Control of Vata will ease your symptoms.

You cannot shake a sugar addiction by trying to go off it cold turkey. You must first replace refined sugar with other Sweet foods like whole grains so that you still get a Sweet "fix" regularly during the day. Ayurvedic supplements can then be used to even out the "spikiness" in your system's response to carbohydrates that is causing the roller-coastering of your blood sugar. Simultaneously, a good diet and good habits will reduce and balance Vata.

ALCOHOL

Alcohol is a sort of super-Sweet substance, one that is metabolized in the same way as sugar. The tremendous Sweet rush which alcohol gives gratifies ahamkara tremendously. Alcoholics are people who find the alcohol-Sweet so superior to other forms of Sweet that they insist on prolonging their experience of it. Alcohol, which is a medicine in small amounts, becomes a poison through overuse. When you ingest alcohol regularly your system creates a balance for itself based on alcohol, and you eventually begin to feel ill if you fail to drink regularly. You are addicted, even if you are not a "classic" alcoholic.

Alcohol dependency is a form of Sweet dependency in which all Three Doshas are disturbed. Small amounts of medicinal wine control Vata-type diseases; larger amounts of alcohol cause Vata diseases. Alcohol, because of its hot, intense taste and smell and its liquid nature, aggravates both Pitta and Kapha. Aggravated Pitta and Kapha then create obstructions to the free movement of Vata and vitiate it. The late stages of alcoholism are purely Vata in nature: shuffling gait, vacant stare, profuse and meaningless speech, severe mood swings, delirium tremens and hallucinations. All these symptoms reflect profound mental and physical "jerkiness" as a result of the irregularities of deranged Vata. Even if you are not frankly alcoholic you will have to calm Vata first and then bring Kapha and Pitta back to normal if you want to eliminate an alcohol habit.

How easy it will be for you to give up alcohol will depend on a number of factors, including the society you live in and your genetic makeup. Recent studies suggest that there are at least two types of genetic sensitivity to alcohol. One type, which need not be too severe, can be passed from father or mother to son or daughter and usually causes alcoholism to develop only after age 25. Another type, which is passed only from father to son, can produce significant brain abnormalities even in those who never drink. Most of these individuals begin drinking early, however, and become alcoholic quickly. Unlike the first type, their behavior is often violent.

People who have been dependent on alcohol and then give it up often trade their addiction to alcohol for addictions to coffee, into which they may pour heaps of sugar, and to Hot, Sour, Salty, Pungent food, like French fries with ketchup and chili sauce. Coffee and chili sauce, both Pungent, replace the Pungent aspect of alcohol's Taste personality. Intensive use of white sugar is the easiest way for the body to get the level of Sweet intake which alcohol has made it accustomed to. Ketchup and other sauces provide the necessary levels of Sour and Salty to force the already overburdened digestive tract to handle the fried food whose heaviness and oil help reduce Vata. The alcoholic body uses these Tastes to preserve its relative balance.

Such people would be better off if they would obtain these various Tastes from more benign foods, simultaneously adding in a little of the Bitter Taste to reduce their intensity requirements. They can obtain Sweetness from whole grains, fruits and fruit juices. Grains provide a regular, stable source of sugar to the blood, and fruit juices like grape or pear can provide quick "fixes" of Sweet when the body demands them. Dates and dried figs strengthen the body and are good sources of intense Sweetness. Pomegranate juice, which provides Sweetness along with Bitterness and Astringency, is therapeutic for Pitta and helps to rejuvenate the system.

The powerfully Sweet juice of the carrot is Hot enough to encourage good digestion and Bitter enough to help reduce the body's need for intense stimulation. The satisfaction and balance that the body receives from carrot juice provides tremendous subliminal satisfaction to the brain. This can compensate to some extent for the lack of pleasurable mental distortion that alcohol provides.

Carrot juice may be consumed alone or, when the liver is especially deranged, beet can be added. Adding the long white daikon radish also helps support weak digestion. Cucumber's Astringency helps reduce intensity craving and soothe inflamed tissues. The superior addition to carrot juice is cilantro, which is Pungent but Cold and flushes heat from both body and mind. Cilantro is one of the best foods there is for reducing anger. When digestion is very weak radish and carrot can be pressure-cooked together into soup with a slice of beet, or these vegetables can be chopped and cooked with mung beans and rice into kichadi, adding fresh cilantro on top before serving.

Coconut is cooling, and its heaviness helps satisfy an alcoholic's craving for heavy food. Fresh coconut milk makes an excellent Sweet unless liver weakness forces a restricted fat intake. It is available in pure form in Asian groceries, or diluted with fruit juice in most health food stores. You can make your own coconut milk if you are fortunate enough to live where fresh coconut is available. Put the shredded flesh of a fresh coconut into a blender, cover it with just enough water to wet it all, blend thoroughly, then strain. Add more cold water and repeat the process. Now add hot water, repeat the process, and discard the coconut remains after this third straining. Mix the three liquids together and, voilà! coconut milk. Mix this with cilantro juice and you have an unbeatable combination for cooling the liver and the Blood.

Alcoholics should mainly use lemon or lime juice as the Sour Tastes in their diets, and should get the Salty Taste from kelp or other seaweed. The amalaki fruit or its powder is the best source of Sourness. Dry ginger is the best source of Pungency, but it should be used carefully to prevent further Pitta disturbance.

Mild laxation, which eliminates accumulated heat and Pitta from the liver, is good purification for someone who has abused alcohol. Bitterness can be provided by herbs such as gentian, barberry, aloe vera, dandelion, punarnava, katuka and bhringaraja, all of which flush toxins from the liver. Dramatic purgation should be avoided, for though it will quickly reduce Pitta its intensity will further aggravate Vata. Since a craving for intensity is one aspect of dependence on alcohol or other drugs, reducing the organism's exposure to intensity is therapeutic.

Physiological balancing removes jerkiness and promotes stability, which in turn assists the mind to right itself and return to normal functioning. People drink alcohol because it inflates ahamkara past her boundaries. These people exist in inflated ahamkara energy, inflated individuality, without regard for spirit, mind or body. The self-disgust and self-pity an alcoholic shows when he or she is sober is a trick that ahamkara plays on the rest of the organism so that it can continue uninterruptedly enjoying its alcohol-food. Alcoholism is, in fact, a disease of ahamkara, of the individuality.

Alcohol is a super-Sweet. No ordinary food can match the intense current of Sweetness that flows with alcohol into the brain. To partially substitute, flood all the senses with Sweet. Let the patient's nose smell Sweet fragrances, like rose, and let his skin feel "Sweet" things, like oil. "Sweet words" should fall into the patient's ears, and "Sweet" surroundings, like life in the country, should meet his eyes. Intense Sweet of all sorts must be provided until the brain is willing and able to scale down its Sweet intake. Otherwise the patient may backslide and return to alcohol, which he or she knows can be relied on to provide Sweetness.

The mind must be strengthened if its faculty of discrimination is to reassert itself. Memory and discrimination can be strengthened with the herb gotu kola, taken as a tea or in capsules washed down with tea of the herb skullcap. Gotu kola is the main ingredient in the Ayurvedic medicine *Brahmi Vati*.

An alcoholic's worst mental problem is weakness of will. The alcohol-dependent ahamkara believes she can live and act independent body, mind or spirit, and is willing to deceive body, mind and spirit as long as she can. To perpetuate her unrestricted indulgence she weakens the individual will power until it can no longer object to her desire to drink. Nothing can be done to remedy this addiction until the individual will power reasserts itself and reestablishes limits for ahamkara. As my teacher Vimalananda put it, "If you want to drink, you must make sure that you are drinking the drink, and that the drink is not drinking you." The alcohol-dependent ahamkara allows drink to consume her whole organism, in return for the false promise of eternal life and vitality that the intoxication of alcohol provides.

Ayurveda recognized alcoholism to be a grave disease more than 3,000 years ago, respecting it for its puissance and its potential to cause harm, and insisting that an alcohol-dependent individual accept outside help to put ahamkara back in her place. Modern-day programs also recognize that the first step in management of any dependency is the recognition that a problem exists. Once ahamkara recognizes that she has gone beyond her limits she opens the door to a new balance for the entire organism.

Chapter Four
Nutrition

The Seven Dhatus

Digested food nourishes both body and mind and provides strength and support for ahamkara and her beloved personality. Ayurveda divides all body tissues into seven classes called *dhatus*, a *dhatu* being anything that provides firmness. Each dhatu satisfies one of the ahamkara's requirements for existence in a human body and "firms up" or "confirms" ahamkara's self-identity with the body. How well your personality fits into your body will determine how well you are able to resist the many aliens who keep challenging your claim to your organism.

The Seven Dhatus are:

Rasa - literally, "sap" or "juice." Rasa represents tissue fluids, including chyle, lymph and blood plasma. Its accessory tissues are breast milk and menstrual blood and its waste product is mucus. Its function is *prinana* (nourishment).

Blood - red blood cells. Its accessory tissues are blood vessels and tendons and its waste is bile. Its function is *jivana* (invigoration).

Flesh - skeletal muscle. Its accessory tissues are ligaments and skin and its wastes are those which accumulate in body orifices: ear wax, snot, navel lint, smegma, and so on. Its function is *lepana* ("plastering" of the skeleton).

Fat - fat in the limbs and torso. Its accessory tissue is omentum and its waste is sweat. *Snehana* (lubrication) is its function.

Bone - all bones. Its accessories are the teeth and its wastes body hair, beard and nails. It provides the body *dharana* (support).

Marrow - anything inside a bone, including red and yellow bone marrow as well as the brain and spinal cord, which are wholly encased in bone. Its accessory tissue is head hair and lachrymal secretions are its wastes. It performs *purana* ("filling" of the bones).

Shukra - male and female sexual fluids. Shukra's tasks are *garbhotpatti* (reproduction) and the production of Ojas, the fluid that generates the aura and controls immunity. It has neither accessory tissues nor waste products.

This scheme is not a fully detailed explanation of human physiology. The rishis were not interested in minute detail; they looked deeper, trying to discover organizing principles. This scheme is an explanation of how ahamkara chooses to clothe herself in flesh.

As long as the dhatus are healthy and well formed, and the wastes are minimal and quickly excreted, ahamkara experiences maximal satisfaction in her incarnation and the individual experiences a deep somatic sense of well-being. When there is inadequate dhatu nutrition ahamkara feels this lack, and her dissatisfaction is transmitted to the consciousness of the individual in question. Digestion and assimilation are essential to an individual's well-being at all levels.

Ayurveda states that each dhatu is formed from the one immediately previous to it, except the accessory tissues, which are only nourished and do not nourish in return. Breast milk and endometrium, for example, are meant for nourishing a child and play no further part in the mother's nutrition. The wastes produced at each stage of dhatu digestion are used in diagnosis, since excess of any waste is indicative of poor digestion at the level of that dhatu.

Most of us would readily accept that ingested food first forms chyle, which then produces red blood cells, which then go to nourish flesh. There our common-sense understanding of the process ceases, however. How can flesh nourish fat, or bone nourish marrow? The answer lies in a re-definition of the word "nourish." These dhatus "nourish" one another by providing metabolic conditions which are conducive to production of the next in line, and by each satisfying a need of ahamkara which allows the next need to be addressed.

For example, if Bone is metabolically unhealthy the body's chemical environment becomes less conducive to proper formation of Marrow, which then is less able to form healthy Shukra. The texts recognize three ways in which this environment can be influenced:

> 1. One dhatu may completely convert itself into another. For example, Rasa provides direct nourishment for the production of Blood. A large part of circulating Rasa is converted into Blood. The Ayurvedic analogy is to the formation of yogurt from milk.

> 2. The dhatu may flow through the body, gradually nourishing the next dhatu in line through a more complicated series of reactions. For example, when Blood nourishes Flesh it flows through many different parts of the body, nourishing Flesh all along the line. The traditional analogy was to the flow of irrigation water through a ditch in a field.

> 3. The dhatu may merely "seed" the next dhatu, by sending hormonal or enzymatic cues to it. This is the way Flesh nourishes Fat and Fat nourishes Bone. It is compared in Ayurveda to the random seeding of a field by a pigeon dropping seeds from its beak.

RASA DHATU

Ahamkara and the dhatus are mutually interdependent. Ahamkara's OK is required before any molecule can be admitted into your body's fellowship, and ahamkara's confidence, which controls its ability to maintain the body's immune defenses, depends upon well-nourished dhatus. The progression of the Seven Dhatus represents the seven stages involved in ahamkara's nourishment. This integration of external, alien material into your internal being is a sensitive operation that begins with the introduction of food into your mouth. As the Tastes alert the brain to the sort of food that has been ingested, the brain directs the digestive process accordingly. As digestion proceeds, material that has passed muster and undergone preliminary conversion is absorbed into the system and begins to circulate. This is Rasa Dhatu.

Rasa has at least two dozen important meanings in Sanskrit, meanings as varied as water, semen, plant sap, and metallic mercury. Rasa Dhatu mainly signifies chyle, blood plasma and lymph, but it also refers to "taste" and "emotion." The fact that Rasa means "taste" suggests that good Rasa Dhatu can be produced only when the ingested food possesses all the Tastes that the organism requires. Those Tastes ensure that the Three Doshas do their jobs properly.

Vata, Pitta and Kapha in turn determine how efficiently digestion and assimilation can occur. Vata controls the movement of nutrients to the cells and wastes from the cells. Insufficient nutrients or excessive wastes interfere with dhatu nutrition. Kapha provides the structures in which these movements occur; disturbed structures mean disturbed transport. Pitta is in charge of conversion of nutrient into body part, and determines how many nutrients will be used and how much waste will be produced.

Rasa Dhatu's special function is "prinana," a word that means nourishment but is derived from a root that signifies romantic love. All bodies live from meal to meal, eternally craving further food. When the body is hungry, each of its cells is hungry. Just as a plant who is withering from lack of attention and water seems to freshen immediately when sprinkled by a thoughtful passerby, so too all of your cells perk up, physically and emotionally, when they receive the "sap" of Rasa Dhatu. Rasa is not sufficient in itself to nourish the whole organism, but it is a promise of better things to come.

Romance is an ephemeral emotion, which projects a potential to provide more. We feel great satisfaction from a glass of juice at the end of a long fast, and great relief from a glass of water after several hours of thirst. But those reactions are really just anticipations of the nourishment your tissues will experience after your digestion operates on that food or water. "Prinana" is the satisfaction you feel when the nourishment first enters your system.

It is called "romantic love" because it is really a waltz of two separate existences—you and the food—who are trying to become sufficiently intimate with one another to unite together. The sense of danger, the exaltation of excitement, the thrill of the unknown and all the other emotions including the lust you feel when you fall in love you also feel, in simpler form, when your body is suffused with the fresh Rasa from a well-digested meal.

If your food is not properly digested, or if it is well digested but improperly assimilated, your ahamkara will feel precisely like the lover whose date stands her up: cheated, used, abused and frustrated. The process of digestion after thorough chewing and swallowing leads ahamkara on to expect a night on the town (good assimilation of healthy Rasa). If ahamkara must wait for hours in growing despair as her corsage wilts, she will take it as an affront to her self-confidence (a weakening of ahamkara's power to project a unified personality). This can lead to self-denigration (weakening of immunity) if it happens too frequently.

The texts list many symptoms that develop when Rasa is disturbed. The most important are "lack of faith" and "lack of taste." "Lack of faith" develops from lack of self-confidence. You can lack faith in yourself or others or both, according to whether your ahamkara concludes that its failure to be nourished derived from its own insufficiency or developed from the malicious intervention of an outside party. Lack of faith can develop into suspicion, which can create barriers against whatever aspect of the outside or inside world has been adjudged by ahamkara to be guilty of treachery.

"Lack of taste" has a twin meaning. Physiologically it indicates a lack of desire for food, which happens when ama is produced in preference to Rasa Dhatu. In such conditions the system recognizes that it must first clear the obstruction to the dhatu nourishment process by digesting ama before it can handle any further nutrition.

Psychologically, "lack of taste" means lack of interest in living, lack of "flavor" for the things in life. An afflicted individual moves about in a perpetual funk, unable to get excited about anything. This is a form of lovesickness: bereft of the love object (Rasa Dhatu) the lover (ahamkara) moves about in a fog, deriving no satisfaction from normal pursuits. The funk is Kapha, the waste product produced at the stage of conversion of food into Rasa. Inefficient conversion produces excessive Kapha, which encourages ama production and creates this lethargy.

If ahamkara's suitor (the food) is exposed as a criminal (ama), a being who actually wishes her harm, he must be kicked out of the house and out of the relationship. Ahamkara must then repair her broken heart (the disorder that ama has created), turn her back on her previous life (avoid certain foods and undergo therapeutic procedures), and wait patiently for a new suitor. Developing mental and emotional health in a personality is next to impossible so long as its physical organism is filled with undigested ama.

BLOOD

When your organism is able to obtain sufficient Rasa, the date between ahamkara and her nourishment takes place, and Rasa has a chance to be converted into Blood. Blood produces "invigoration," that rush of vitality that makes us feel the full vibrancy of life. Some of the sense of danger evaporates as ahamkara gets to know her date and finds him exciting and stimulating. She is fascinated by him—he has "got into her blood"—and she begins to think of him as a potentially fit mate for her. Hope and anticipation invigorate her.

When Rasa is not well digested Blood is insufficiently produced and Pitta, the waste product at this stage, is overproduced. Like Blood, Pitta is a hot, intense influence. But Pitta cannot perform Blood's invigoration function. Pitta can only heat up the organism, resulting in increased anger (at the love object for refusing to submit to domination by ahamkara) and jealousy (lest any other ahamkara dare to try to snatch the roving love object away). "Hot-blooded lovers" have ample Rasa for romance or lust but too much scorching Pitta in their blood, energy that can lead to violence as it exits the individual.

FLESH

When Blood is healthy and well formed it nourishes Flesh, whose job is "plastering," covering of the skeleton and internal organs so that they are not exposed to the outside. The wastes produced at this stage are wastes that develop in and sometimes occlude body orifices. Flesh also provides a preliminary barrier between the "you" of your organism and the "not-you" of the external world. Your muscle fibers provide you a sense of security; they are the bricks and stones of your body's fortifications against attack from without.

At the level of Flesh our couple—the ahamkara and her food—have decided to go steady. He commits to defending her as his against all challenges; she now has a protector, a "bodyguard," to shelter her from the world. An ahamkara who lacks sufficient healthy Flesh feels naked and defenseless, uncovered to the world, open to external influences in spite of romance and invigoration. Body builders who turn away from all other human pursuits in order to magnify their muscles are often insecure individuals who use those muscles to insulate themselves from the need to interact substantively with anyone on the outside.

FAT

Well-nourished Flesh feeds Fat, whose function is "sneha," which literally means unctuousness. Sneha also means love, though love of a different sort from prinana. Sneha is a bonded, secure love relationship, like that which exists between mother and child or husband and wife. Just as loving partners snuggle and cuddle together for warmth, fat "snuggles" our bodies and provides us warm, satisfying love. Ahamkara and her food have finally tied the knot and are now wed to one another, for better or for worse. Fat, and to some extent Flesh as well, provide us with that sublime satisfaction that a sound sleeper receives from a warm quilt on a cold night.

Fat and its waste product sweat both help maintain the body's internal temperature. Fat insulates us to hold heat in, and sweat radiates heat away. A human whose Fat is insufficient is perpetually physically and emotionally cold, lacking that thermal insulation which Fat provides. This coldness inspires such an individual to seek increased physical and mental nourishment to nourish Fat and achieve the warm, satisfying love it can give. Remember the cold-blooded Cassius and his "lean and hungry look," who pursued his ends with little concern for the means he used. Cassius searched for gratification, not for love, as does anyone who enjoys lust, invigoration and physical security while assiduously avoiding sincere emotional commitment. It is possible that the anorexic look which is so popular in fashion today is partly derived from the drive for independence and rootlessness which breaks bonds and restrictive relationships and displays itself psychosomatically as a near-pathological aversion to Fat/commitment.

Some people who despair of ever locating a bonded love relationship with another human turn to the solace that food can provide and accumulate an extreme overabundance of Fat. Such warm-hearted people simply lack that loving life-partner or that stable family situation which could act as an object for their affection. The satisfaction an obese individual feels in being fat is real and perceptible to ahamkara, and the likelihood of successful, permanent weight loss in such people is low until ahamkara is redirected and becomes willing to relinquish the "security blanket" to which she clings. This affection must be directed at other objects, perhaps externally to community service activities or internally to spiritual development. Obesity is neither a simple psychological problem nor a simple problem of nutrition. It is a problem of psychological nutrition.

BONE

Healthy Fat makes for healthy Bone, whose job is "support." Bone makes it possible for us to move in the world. Without our bony skeletons we would all lie limply on the floor like jellyfish. The bones and joints are closely connected with the mind's ability to express itself, since proficiency of expression is a function of ability to move. Bone is "supportive" as well as "supporting"; it allows us to project our own identities out into the world in the same way that its wastes—body hair, beard and nails—grow and project themselves from the interior into the exterior. When support is lacking we can derive only limited satisfaction from gratification, invigoration, security and commitment.

Though the previous four dhatus perfuse the whole organism they focus on its periphery: the limbs, skin and body wall. Bone marks a shift in emphasis, for now food begins to flow deeply into the organism's interior, into its center. Now that ahamkara has protected her ability to maintain her internal integrity she must stabilize her ability to present a coherent, unified face to the world. Weak Bone reduces ahamkara's support for her external projection. Think of the epithet "spineless wonder" and you have a mental picture of the effect of unhealthy Bone on an individual. Healthy Bone allows ahamkara to concretize her personality and establish firm personal parameters.

MARROW

Bone produces Marrow. Marrow is anything that is entirely encased in bone, including the fatty yellow bone marrow, the blood-forming red bone marrow, and the brain and spinal cord. Note that although Marrow physically produces Blood, Blood is identified in Ayurveda with the liver, which modern medicine knows to be the controller of blood production, if not its actual site. Ayurveda is interested in root causes.

The function of Marrow is "filling." Bone and the colon enjoy a mutual affinity, both being prone to accumulation of Vata as a result of being hollow. When Bone is well "filled" with Marrow it retains little empty space in which Vata can accumulate. On the mental plane healthy Marrow prevents emptiness of mind. Already the food has provided the ahamkara a firm foundation against which to brace while projecting; any good spouse would do this. Now the food dives deeper into the depths of the organism and pools itself inside the Bony bastions which ahamkara has created for it. As Marrow it acts as an energy-storage medium, something like a bank of capacitors or batteries: a pool of passive, easily available power.

The mere ability to project your personality into the world is insufficient for health, even when you feel gratified, invigorated, secure, loved and confident. Unless there is something of value present in your personality which you can project, you are hollow, your "headpiece filled with straw," your words "full of sound and fury and signifying nothing." This disease, which is very prevalent today, reflects the world's generally poor state of dhatu nutrition. It is diagnosable from the eyes, which are the single most significant projector of the personality into the environment.

Healthy Marrow gives the eyes a clear, strong sheen that radiates calm light just like a lamp flame in a quiet place radiates silent, tranquil light. Dull, lifeless eyes indicate weak Marrow. In some terminal diseases, like galloping consumption, the eyes become feverishly bright toward the end. This does not indicate health, of course; it shows that the organism has marshaled its last fading reserves of strength and is using them to project its personality bravely outwards until the end. The body burns its own tissues to provide the light ahamkara needs to project herself outward through her windows on the world, the eyes.

Marrow is prone to inadequate nutrition, even when the rest of the body is healthy, because of the drying, roughening and destabilizing effects of Vata. Since Bone is one of the chief seats of Vata and Marrow is derived from Bone, Vata increase in Bone will play havoc with Marrow's nourishment. Marrow that has been thus weakened can then disturb the rest of the organism, via Bone. Some empty-Marrow individuals can project their personalities into the world and influence others with great ease. Though they seem forceful and persuasive there is no substance to their projection. It is all so much "hot air," being a product of Vata. Eventually this Vata disturbance works its way into Bone, and the bloated balloon of the inflated, aggrandized personality finally bursts. Then all the hot air whooshes out leaving the individual crumpled in a heap on the ground, depleted in both Bone and Marrow.

SHUKRA AND OJAS

Properly nourished Marrow goes to nourish *Shukra*, which is the collective word for all secretions involved in reproduction. The food has now been transformed into a substance that can unite with ahamkara. Shukra's functions are creation and creativity. It can be used for procreation (the production of children) or for the production of artistic or intellectual creations. Shukra's job is to act as a matrix through which new creations can manifest on our plane of existence. It is the clay which creativity shapes into forms.

Weak Shukra means weak creativity. Afflicted individuals may seemingly have it all. They may be gratified, invigorated, secure and loved, may be able to project themselves cogently and coherently into their environment, and may have plenty to offer. Without strong Shukra, though, they will not be able to consummate any productive arrangement or exert any lasting effect on the flow of events. A child is a lasting effect; so is a new corporation, a sheaf of music, or an amended law. Shukra controls an individual's ability to make a mark on the slate of the world.

When ahamkara couples excitedly and expansively with Shukra it tends to lose control of the creative energy it arouses. This creativity then flows out of the body into another body via the sex act, or into some project or enterprise via the voice or hands. When ahamkara can couple with Shukra calmly and collectedly, a new substance called Ojas is created. Properly tended Ojas will remain within the body, solidifying the link between our physical, mental and spiritual existences.

All forms of physical and mental indigestion damage Ojas and encourage ama formation. Indigestion is easiest to deal with when it is limited to the digestive tract. Once it moves into the dhatus, where it disrupts the ahamkara's ability to nourish herself, managing ama becomes much more complicated. When ama blocks dhatu nutrition in your digestive tract your life first loses its zest as Rasa becomes malnourished and polluted with Kapha. Then Pitta-polluted Blood saps your vitality, malnourished Flesh strips you of your security, and each dhatu in turn is weakened until Ojas, the foundation of your immunity, is starved into dysfunction. Mind pollutes body by forcing it into unhealthy activities, and body pollutes mind by producing ama and starving the organism of Ojas. Mind and body are concurrently and inherently joined.

Obesity

Obesity is an appropriate illustration of the interaction between mind and body and its implications for the dhatus and for ahamkara. Obesity, like gout and diabetes, is classified in Ayurveda as one of the "diseases of affluence." Affluence is not restricted to the rich; every one of us who has resources to waste is affluent. Affluence, or rather the affluent state of mind that believes it can waste with abandon, is the real disease; obesity, gout and diabetes are only its symptoms.

Most residents of the affluent countries of the West feel "affluent," and it is not surprising that most of us Westerners need to lose some weight. In fact, two of every three adults in the United States are overweight. In 1997 a researcher at Harvard University reported that roughly one of every five Americans is obese—about 53 million people—and that 300,000 people die each year in our country from obesity. Mass advertising exhorts us to consume continuously, since constant consumption is the mechanism by which our affluence has been obtained, and we do. An Ayurvedic text comments: "Boredom, mindless entertainment, continuous eating, and oversleeping: these will fatten you up just like a hog." Most of us have experienced the truth of this saying during the holidays, when liberated from drudgery we stuff ourselves like pigs and then watch TV until we become so bored and indolent that we fall asleep. This is an infallible way to gain weight, and if repeated regularly it can lead to obesity.

But our popular culture worships thinness. One of the most malignant of the several epidemics that is surging through the West today is that of *dysmorphophobia*, the "fear of having a misshapen body." Repeated exposure from a young age to our ideal of beauty—thin, leggy, nearly hipless—teaches girls and young women (and their mothers) to evaluate their worth in terms of their appearance. Recent surveys suggest that more than 80% of fourth graders in California have already been on a diet and that nationally 40% of girls age 9 and 10 have tried to lose weight. 70% of teenage girls in America diet; others exercise so fanatically that their puberty maybe delayed or they may stop menstruating for months at a time. Some even develop osteoporosis when they become so over-conditioned that their total body fat falls beneath the minimum level that the body needs to produce its hormones.

Extreme dieting can mutate into anorexia, bulimia and binge eating, addictive behaviors which now affect seven million women and one million men in the United States. An estimated 20% of U.S. college women have eating disorders, and recent studies suggest that increasing numbers of college men are now developing dysfunctional eating patterns and outright eating disorders.

Other cultures, like that of India, have an entirely different concept of beauty than do we. Almost no one in India, no matter how wealthy, believes that thin is beautiful. Every hero and heroine of the Indian silver screen is plump. The incidence of eating disorders in India and in other developing countries is negligible (except among the Westernized élites) because people there openly enjoy the variety of ahamkara-gratification that both society and Fat provide. Our culture, though, prizes individuality over bonding, and eating disorders have accordingly become epidemic here.

The media plays an important part in this pathology. We are bombarded daily with conflicting suggestions: eat constantly and feel affluent, but never gain weight! It is a wonder that even more of us have not been driven insane by such incongruous suggestions. Many of us who have not lost our senses from this inconsistency have become neurotic, though, and neurosis is enough to cause a person to become either obese or anorexic. Food neuroses develop from the interplay of the suppression of these conflicting emotions and the influence of internal chemical imbalances. Internal confusion encourages us to recede further into affluence, which compounds the problem. Excess weight and emotional trauma entwine with one another to create a problem that can be very resistant to solution.

Some people are better able than others to satisfy the paradoxical cultural requirements of our society. Variations in ability to lose weight occur because of what some modern scientists call the "fat setpoint," the level of fat your body tries to maintain because it functions best at that level. The main influence on this "setpoint"—let us call it instead your "fat ideal"—is your genetics, acting through your personal constitution. V people burn food quickly and have to intensively overeat in order to become obese. VP people are almost this lucky, and P people can usually lose any weight they might temporarily gain. VK people are slow to gain weight and equally slow to lose it. PK and K people always seem to have some extra poundage somewhere that they want to get rid of no matter how little they eat.

Another critical influence occurs during infancy when the number of fat cells you have is finalized. These fat cells once formed are permanent residents of your body. When you lose weight the amount of fat within each one is reduced, but the cells themselves never disappear. Children who are overfed poor diets are sure to develop a large number of fat cells, and until the ends of their lives they will find it easy to gain weight and difficult to take it off again. Fat babies make for fat adults.

Attitude also counts. Fear tends to refuse to allow nutrients into the system, which is why V people often have difficulty gaining weight. However, anyone who overeats to calm fear will eventually gain weight. Anger burns away nutrients, which is how P people may escape obesity despite their strong hunger, but anyone who overeats specifically to cool anger eventually gains weight. K people tend to hold weight on anyway, and anyone who overeats to gratify a need for Fat-type bonded love (a Kapha-mediated reason) is sure to gain weight. People who, filled with Bitterness due to intense frustration, choose to obtain life's Sweetness through food may become addicted to the pleasures of eating and may become obese. Individual reasons for obesity vary, but all of them involve the determination of ahamkara to hold tenaciously to her beloved Fat, the dhatu that provides reliable, steady love and warmth.

No diet, however strict, can change this. Loneliness is worse for you than a high-fat diet when you are trying to lose weight. Most strict diets are actually self-defeating, for they manifest from an attitude of self-hatred, of disgust for the fat and for the self whose weakness allowed the fat to accumulate. This attitude leads to a desire to starve the body in order to punish the mind. The body feels starved during any crash diet, and because it does not like to be starved it acts on its own to preserve its highest energy tissue by lowering its metabolic rate, which burns fat more slowly. It also tends to first burn off those tissues that are not immediately needed. Anyone who diets but does not exercise will therefore lose lean tissue first, since it is not being regularly used.

Hunger pangs increase as the body tries to force the mind to eat more and satisfy its hunger. This affects junk food addicts worst, since their bodies have been emptied of many essential nutrients that their bodies experience severe hunger for when dieting. Moreover, when dieters go back to their normal eating habits at the end of a diet they burn off less calories and store more fat than they did previously. Their metabolic rates have dropped, and their bodies are now wary of starvation and want to store even more just in case such an episode should be repeated. Crash dieting therefore increases the body's fat ideal, and makes you fatter!

The psychological effects of crash dieting are even more pernicious. Both starving people and dieters dream and fantasize about food, and both suffer from anxiety and depression, all from the physical stress of having to live below the body's desired fat ideal. The body and mind of a dieter are at daggers drawn with one another. When the organism can no longer withstand the body's incessant demands for food it cheats on its diet. The mind's first reaction is then to binge, because "I've already gone off my diet, so why not?" After the binge guilt rears up, as the mind realizes that its temporary indulgence in food has damaged its physical self-image. To remedy this the dieter returns to penance and starts back down the road to starvation, little knowing that such erratic behavior inexorably drives up your fat ideal as it aggravates Vata.

Even resisting temptation can be hazardous to your weight. Every dieter who lusts after a luscious dessert sends a message to the brain that new and tasty morsels are about to be consumed. This makes the mouth water and the digestive juices start to flow, and signals the body's insulin to remove some sugar from the general circulation to make way for the new sugar which will soon be flooding the blood. The body stores this sugar as fat.

Lowered blood sugar increases the appetite. Whenever you crave a tempting dessert but restrain yourself from eating it you add a little fat at the moment of craving. When you next eat you will eat more than you would normally have eaten, for your mental lust for the dessert has lowered your blood sugar and increased both your physical appetite for carbohydrate and your mental appetite for Sweet. Added body fat increases insulin production, which causes more and more fat to be deposited at each episode. You really can gain weight just by looking at a tasty pastry!

Eventually excess fat makes your insulin less sensitive to your blood sugar level, because the body resists laying down any more fat after it passes its preferred ideal. Then your blood sugar begins to increase above normal, which means diabetes. When the tissues lose their ability to use insulin the muscles lose access to their regular supply of sugar fuel. Feeling starved, they will send persistent demands to the brain for more food, thus deepening the downward spiral of malnutrition and damaging ahamkara further. Overnourishment of a dhatu is as bad or worse than undernourishment.

Most cases of diabetes that develop in this way do not require insulin for treatment. Weight loss if often enough to return insulin function to normal and ensure that the tissues are again well fed. Diabetes, like all "diseases of affluence," responds well to austerity.

Gaining Weight

Austerity is precisely the wrong prescription for those people who either have never been able to gain weight or have dieted and exercised themselves into emaciation. First their Rasa Dhatu dries out, and then their other dhatus follow suit. Their bodies retreat into a continual state of hunger and thirst, compounding Vata excess with deficiency of Prana. Breathing difficulties are common in such people, as is in extreme cases damage to the internal organs.

The treatment of emaciation is the treatment of Vata, according to the verse mentioned above: "Boredom, mindless entertainment, continuous eating, and oversleeping: these will fatten you up just like a hog." Not boredom, of course, but relaxation, reduction in stress and responsibility, abatement of the need to achieve the anorexic "ideal." Not "mindless entertainment" but sufficient recreation to balance any overachieving tendency, combined with Yoga to promote mental peace and regular massage with ample oil. Mild exercise is essential, to encourage the body to gradually reset its fat ideal. Continuous eating should take the form of four or five small meals each day. Adequate, restful sleep, during the Kapha and Pitta portions of the night, combined with a half-hour nap most afternoons. These simple lifestyle changes are sometimes sufficient to fatten up a thin person.

Vardhamana Pippali Rasayana is one simple practice that can facilitate weight gain in many people. It involves mixing on the first morning one cup of milk with half a cup of water, a teaspoon of maple syrup or freeze-dried sugar cane juice and one fruit of long pepper (*Piper longum*). Boil this down to one cup, strain, and drink, chewing up the boiled long pepper if you so desire. Next morning use two long pepper fruits, three on the third morning, and so on, up to twenty-one. On the twenty-second day take twenty fruits, nineteen fruits on the twenty-third day, and so on, decreasing by one each day until you are back down to zero. This practice aims to reawaken the digestive fire and rejuvenate Rasa Dhatu, without whose participation no weight gain will last.

Losing Weight

Emaciation still takes a back seat in importance in our society to obesity. Permanent weight loss occurs only when the body's fat ideal is lowered. The amphetamines and other chemicals in prescription diet pills and the nicotine in tobacco can temporarily lower your fat ideal, but these effects will last for only so long as you use the drug. You are bound to gain weight again as soon as you stop smoking or quit swallowing the pills. Besides, drugs are addictive; nicotine is in fact even more addictive than heroin.

Drugs lower the body's fat ideal by speeding up the organism, making both body and brain work faster. Speed of any sort increases Vata, which makes both body and mind crave increased Sweet for balance. Nicotine and diet pills provide a certain intense Sweet to the brain but not to the body. When the drug is removed the accumulated physical craving of the tissues for nutrition forces the individual to eat excessively, leading to guilt at indiscipline, further dramatic attempts to lose weight, and a generalized Vata increase which further unbalances the body and deepens the neurosis.

Ayurveda believes in speeding up the organism in healthy, natural ways, controlling Vata while relieving the system of excess Kapha. Ayurveda uses exercise, supplements, and light, non-Kapha-producing foods in a process that is slower than most dieters would prefer. In weight loss, as in all other aspects of medicine, haste makes waste.

If you are overweight and suffer from all or most of the following symptoms, you urgently need to reduce your poundage under competent professional guidance:

- Pendulous belly, breasts and buttocks
- Puffing and panting for breath even on mild exertion
- Profuse perspiration even when it is not hot
- Excess thirst, especially at night
- Intense food cravings
- Prolonged but unsatisfying sleep
- Unpleasant body odor
- Inflammation where skin folds rub against one another
- Generalized body ache
- Loss of sexual appetite
- Lack of zeal or enthusiasm for living

If you do **not** suffer from most of these symptoms you should **not** attempt severe dieting or other heroic attempts to lose weight. You should focus instead on bringing yourself into balance, taking whatever guidance you need to ensure that you succeed. Some people are strong-willed enough to succeed at redefining themselves on their own, but most people require some external support when healing, particularly when they are trying to relinquish an addiction to food. It might be a spouse, a close friend, or a group of individuals who all suffer from the same problem, but it must be a source of support in which you can place your complete trust, allowing your actions to be guided as you accept advice on how to proceed. You should be prepared to accept any good assistance that you may receive.

You cannot be in any hurry if you want to make your weight loss permanent. Your body needs time to readjust itself and lower its fat ideal, and until that ideal drops your weight will not. Some things, like the development of children in the womb, simply cannot be rushed. In this situation you are trying to create an entirely new you.

Carl Jung taught that the thing the cures a neurosis must be as real and convincing as the neurosis itself, and this is particularly true when you are working with the self-image that ahamkara has set for herself. A new body silhouette and a new outlook on life require profound personality alterations, and slow progress permits your mind to adjust itself to the new persona. Besides, quick weight loss stresses the body as toxins that are trapped in the tissues are liberated faster than the body's waste disposal systems can handle them. It also stresses ahamkara, who becomes alarmed when the security of Fat is eliminated before other sources of secure, bonded love can be developed.

Affluence of mind is the true cause of obesity. Your transformation begins when you desist from the boredom which causes you to eat because you feel you have nothing better to do. Being so disgusted with yourself that you eat from sorrow at your seeming inability to change is also a form of affluence. Your goal should be to transform yourself, not to lose weight. Reducing your weight is a part of self-transformation that occurs automatically.

Spring is the best time to begin your bodily renovation. Everything is renewed in spring, and the warmth of spring and the heat of summer will help melt your fat and reset your ideal. Any time is a good time to begin, though, even if it is beginning again. Never give up; even if you fail 100 times begin again the 101st. Every attempt will benefit you, if it is sincere. Eventually you are bound to succeed.

There is no permanent weight loss without regular exercise. People who exercise four or five times a week lose weight at least three times faster than those who exercise only thrice a week. Exercise once or twice a week is insufficient to alter your fat ideal. Moderate, sustained exercise is better than vigorous exertion. Even a brisk walk for half an hour is sufficient, if it is brisk enough. Strenuous massage acts as a passive exercise that moves the muscles and releases the endorphins. However it suits you, you must get your body moving.

When your body moves so will your breath. You receive Prana, the life force, from both air and food. Your system will feel less hunger if your breathing is good, for good breathing permits the body to rely less on food for its Prana. Whenever you feel hungry first sit down and take ten deep breaths. If you are still hungry afterwards you can eat, but most of the time you will find that your hunger has faded.

Oversleeping is a significant cause of overweight. To reduce your sleep go to bed each night at the same time and wake up each morning at the same time. If you go to sleep earlier than usual one day you must arise earlier than usual the next morning. Try to arise half an hour before dawn, or at least by 6 a.m. After a month of regularizing your sleep pattern, reduce your total period of sleep by half an hour. Most people find it easiest to go to sleep a half-hour later each night than to get up a half-hour earlier each morning. Reduce your sleep half an hour each month until you reach your minimum. Everyone has a different minimum. Six hours is good for most of us, but some of us need seven or eight. Except during illness no one should sleep longer than eight hours a night.

If you find you simply cannot reduce your sleep by these means then wake yourself in the middle of the night, after a minimum of four hours of sleep, and get out of bed. Walk around, sit and read, do anything except eat. Stay awake for at least half an hour, and then return to sleep. This breaking up of the soundness of your sleep will help reduce your sleep habit without affecting your rest. Never sleep during the day when you are trying to lose weight.

Please eat according to the suggestions made in the chapter on food, and fast once a week according to your prakriti. Also, increase your eating awareness. Much unnecessary eating is done unconsciously. Some people keep a journal, writing down either before or after the meal a list of foods consumed. Others read their menu into a tape recorder. Still others count to three before each mouthful is eaten. Whatever system you adopt, no matter how silly it may seem, make sure that it requires you to be aware of each substance at every meal. Awareness is the key to personal transformation.

Be sure to chew thoroughly. Chewing releases flavor from food, and since fat people are usually addicted to flavor thorough chewing will produce more satisfaction from less food. The act of chewing itself helps satisfy food cravings, and one way to avoid eating when you crave jaw stimulation is to chew beeswax or sugarless gum. To achieve greater sensory pleasure eat each food article separately. Use one-pot meals only if you need them to control Vata. Refrain from daydreaming or fantasizing about food; don't forget that lusting after tasty morsels actually adds to your fat. Take a walk, chew your beeswax, or drink some herbal tea when your imagination becomes overactive.

Reward yourself regularly for good behavior. Permit yourself indulgences in other sensory areas when you achieve success at disciplining your food intake. Make sure that your intake of Sweet through your other senses is sufficient to make up for the Sweet that used to come to you through your tongue. Never punish yourself for backsliding. Punishment for failure reduces hope and confidence for eventual success, reinforces guilt, and weakens the new self-image you are trying to create for yourself. Whenever and whatever you eat, enjoy your food!

If you can observe no other restriction at least do not eat too fast or too often.

All food that increases Kapha tends to increase weight. Likewise, all food that helps control Kapha discourages weight gain. You should especially avoid the following foods:

> Beef and pork; butter, cheese, ice cream, sour cream; wheat and wheat products; white sugar and all products containing white sugar; alcoholic beverages; fried foods of any sort; junk food and fast food; all excessively Sour or Salty foods like pickles.

Merely going on an anti-Kapha diet when you want to lose weight may be entirely inappropriate if you are a V person who needs Kapha-promoting food to maintain balance. It would best for you to stabilize your diet first after removing all the objectionable foods above. Unless your Doshas are balanced your dhatus, including Fat, will never become healthy.

Change your diet gradually. Do not salt your food at all; if you want the Salty Taste, use "light" salt, kelp powder, or liquid amino-acid preparations (unless you are sensitive to MSG!). Limit your use of sweeteners, but allow yourself regular use of honey (except in cooking). Honey has a mild fat-reducing effect. Take fiber (like bran or psyllium seed husk) whenever you sweets; fiber helps the body balance its response to Sweet. Though fruit is Sweet its fiber usually does not permit its sugars to be absorbed too quickly. The fiber in whole grains also protects against exaggerated blood sugar levels.

While high-protein diets may promote quick weight loss they will also create extra wastes and promote mental overactivity. A high-carbohydrate diet, such as one that contains large amounts of whole grains, tends to make its consumer feel more relaxed and "mellow." You will lose weight more enjoyably and more comfortably if you eat a reasonable amount of carbohydrate. Also, fat requires carbohydrate to burn, so trying to deny yourself all carbohydrate while you live on protein and vegetables makes the weight loss more difficult and less certain.

As you feel it is safe and sensible to do so, reduce the quantity of food that you eat. Keeping your largest meal at midday, reduce the amounts that you eat in the morning and the afternoon. Make a sustained effort not to eat after sunset. As you reduce your food quantity your stomach will shrink little by little and you will soon find your capacity for food reduced. Excessive eating is often more a problem with overweight V and P types than it is with overweight Ks, whose bodies tend to hang on to excess pounds even if they do not overeat.

Eliminate all cold food and drink. You should eat nothing that is refrigerator cold. Fat is the body's insulation and increases naturally when the body is subjected to cold. Continuous exposure to cold food and drink, and even to air conditioning, convinces the body that it should add extra insulation, so up goes the fat ideal. Exercise, which helps heat the body, reduces its need for insulation.

Reduce your overall water intake as you reduce the salt in your diet. You should always drink when you are physically thirsty, but you do not necessarily need the 6 to 8 glasses of water daily that some "nutritional authorities" advocate. Warm water or hot herbal teas help melt fat away. Even better is honey and lemon in warm water, with a pinch of black pepper powder.

When you are fed up with all these restrictions, go out and binge without guilt, preferably on healthful foods, and then forget about it. Cravings for your old food friends are only panic reactions of your body or mind. If you reassure your self with familiar food that you are not trying to starve it to death your craving to binge will become less and less frequent.

It may be wise to take vitamin and mineral supplements during this period of transition to ensure that your body does not lack any nutrients. Ayurvedic herbal preparations may also help. Ayurvedic supplements can mobilize and eliminate fat from the body, and can help reduce your fat ideal. These products are not appetite suppressants; they are substances that encourage permanent metabolic change. They synergize dietary control and exercise to make excess fat swiftly disappear, and encourage it to stay away once it is gone.

Though any Bitter, Pungent or Astringent food, herb or mineral will exert some weight-reducing effect some are clearly more active than others are. A few active herbs are barberry, black pepper, gentian, golden seal, gotu kola, red raspberry leaves, saffron and turmeric. Some of the Ayurvedic compounds that are prescribed in India for weight reduction include:

> The powder called *Triphala* ("three fruits"), especially when it is combined with *Trikatu* ("three pungents"), a mixture of equal parts of powdered ginger, black pepper and *pippali* (long pepper or *Piper longu*m).

> The liver purifier *Arogya Vardhini*.

Chandra Prabha, a compound that includes a form of mineral pitch called *Shilajit.*

Guggulu (Commiphora mukul), a gum closely related to myrrh. Guggulu has been used successfully in India to treat such diseases as hepatitis and myocardial necrosis. It helps reduce blood cholesterol, is an emmenagogue and analgesic, and seems to show some anti-fertility activity. The guggulu formula most used to reduce fat is *Triphala Guggulu.*

Triphala Guggulu's ingredients are Triphala, Trikatu and guggulu. This mixture is mixed with strong Triphala tea and rubbed in a mortar and pestle until it is dry, whereupon small pills are made. Triphala purifies the body of old ama trapped in the Fat; Trikatu helps lower the body's fat ideal; and guggulu actually "scrapes" Fat away from the other tissues. Triphala Guggulu should be taken with warm water or tea of dry ginger to facilitate its fat-scraping action.

Many people suffer from the peculiar notion that if one pill works well ten should work ten times as well. Continued use of substantial overdoses of guggulu over many months can cause Doshas to accumulate in the lungs and liver. Overuse of guggulu can promote dryness of mouth or body, impotence, darkness of vision, emaciation, faintness, and looseness of the limbs. Fortunately the spice saffron can alleviate guggulu-caused symptoms. The same precautions apply to the use of myrrh. These side-effects occur only when the system becomes addicted to the presence of guggulu and is not due to any toxicity on guggulu's part.

All Ayurvedic preparations work better once you have purified your system. In addition to traditional Ayurvedic purifications it is good to use castor oil before you begin your use of guggulu. If you are at least 40 pounds heavier than your ideal weight you may for six weeks take 1 Tbsp. of castor oil each morning after arising and wash it down with a strong cup of tea of dry ginger. This will not produce a laxative effect but will start the scraping action on Fat. You may also use a gland-balancing compound like Tikta for at least a month before beginning with Triphala Guggulu to enhance its effect.

An ideal weight for you is one that is appropriate for your constitution, which means that K types can forget about achieving the anorexic magazine model look. Even though Ayurveda states that it is better to be too thin than too fat, remember that insufficient Fat weakens ahamkara and damages immunity. Fat is an essential dhatu; it is good for you, in the proper amount. Hatred of your fat is self-hatred, a corrosive emotion that can weaken ahamkara yet further. Forget about Fat; think only about recreating yourself.

Chapter Five
Routine

Recipes make cooking easier. Healthful habits are part of the recipe for recreating yourself. When your dhatus are in flux ahamkara is less able to firmly identify with the body, which increases opportunities for illness to develop. Ayurveda believes that routine discipline for body and mind actively strengthens immunity by providing a foundation upon which ahamkara can build a new you.

The Rishis who manifested Ayurveda determined long ago which habits were desirable and which should be avoided, and prepared daily and seasonal routines for people of varying prakritis to follow for health maintenance. V people especially need routine because they are so innately irregular. V types find it very hard to stick to any routine for any length of time. K types love routine, but often their routines are unhealthy. They find as much difficulty in eliminating bad habits as Vs do in adding good ones. P types can add or remove habits almost at will, but they may have difficulty distinguishing between good and bad habits.

Many people are convinced that they have no time to allot to creating and following good habits. My teacher Vimalananda used to say, "Westerners wear their gods on their wrists." By this he meant that we allow an artificial, arrhythmic version of time to regulate our lives. All organisms require rhythm for proper functioning, but most of us ignore the natural internal and external rhythms that secretly influence us. We try instead to create our own, unnatural time. Our dedication to arbitrary schedules robs us of our natural rhythms and weakens our ability to adapt to stresses. Fortunately, introducing additional routine into our lives can regenerate these rhythms. The human organism loves routine and thrives when it is fed, exercised and rested regularly.

The need for discipline with regard to indulgence in food, sleep and sex is especially strong. Whatever your constitution, food, sleep and sex are the Three Pillars of your life, the three activities which when strong support the house which is your body. When they are weakened by misuse your house collapses. Since your health depends upon the support it receives from these Three Pillars, good food, sleep and sex habits are essential if you want to make a success of your life.

The Three Pillars represent digestion, rest and creativity. Food is that which the body digests, which nourishes your organism. Overindulgence in food mainly aggravates Pitta and leads to improper physical and mental digestion. Sleep is that which forces the mind to rest from its perpetual outward projection, and allows your personal identity to consolidate its control over your whole organism. Overindulgence in sleep mainly aggravates Kapha and dulls the dynamism of body and mind. Sex is that which procreates and allows you to temporarily merge with another being. Overindulgence in sex mainly aggravates Vata and weakens your creativity and ability to communicate.

Properly consumed and digested food provides you the energy you require for creation, the projection of the uniqueness of your individuality into the environment. You may project your energy into matter to create an art form or a balance sheet, or you may dissipate it by projecting it into unproductive activities like watching TV. If during the day you fail to either create with your energy or dissipate it you will be tempted at night to project that energy into another human being during the sex act. The energy may be used to create another human form or to create satisfaction in your partner, or it may simply be dissipated. After such transmission you rest from your craving to project and express yourself by entering the state of rest known as sleep, which prepares you for the next day's energy intake and expenditure. Digestion, creation, and rest are daily essentials for every healthy individual of any constitution. Health demands that you enjoy just enough food, sleep and sex, no more and no less.

Most of us are too busy to follow all the suggestions listed in this chapter. Try incorporating into your daily routine whatever you find useful for your own needs and aims from among these proposals. A good routine will improve your health, enhance your ability to perform your duties and accumulate possessions, and aid you in the fulfillment of your legitimate desires.

Daily Routine

One of the most important goals of a good morning routine is to prepare you to consume your next meal by purifying your organism of its wastes. You must eliminate the refuse from the previous day before you add new fuel to your system, just as you would remove the ashes from a fireplace before making a new fire there. To minimize your wastes is to maximize your efficiency. Wastes include urine, feces, sweat; all filth which accumulates on the sense organs; and all mental wastes like emotions, obsessions, and delusions. Salient points in Ayurveda's proposed daily routine include:

ARISING

Awaking before sunrise permits the body to begin to synchronize itself to the rhythm of the sun. Also, Vata, whose qualities of lightness and irregularity do not encourage good sound sleep, rules the last portion of the night. Since Vata is also involved in elimination, the pre-dawn period is the best time to try to eliminate the body's physical and mental wastes. Proper elimination also helps remove the Kapha that naturally accumulates overnight.

Vata's lightness also encourages good meditation. Sleep is a kind of death, a partial dissociation of the mind and spirit from the body. The sun's magnanimity in giving life by burning its own being to provide us with light and heat has induced many cultures to worship the sun as a deity. Everyone should rise early and marvel a few moments over the miracle of existence which is about to begin again, allowing this miracle to instill a deep-felt reverence for all life in the core of your being. Early morning is a good time to request Nature to maintain and amplify your own harmony during the day so that you will interact harmoniously with everyone and everything you encounter.

WASTES

Defecation once or twice daily is best. Three or more times a day unnecessarily increases Vata, the force which must expel the wastes, and encourages food to move through the gut too fast to be properly absorbed. Defecating immediately after a meal should not be encouraged, though it is wise to urinate immediately after each meal. Always clench your teeth tightly when voiding either urine or feces, to prevent Vata from loosening them.

Examine your urine and feces each morning and decide if they are healthy. Any disturbance in your wastes indicates poor digestion, and signs like undigested food in your feces betray the presence of ama. You should try to remedy this situation before the imbalance has an opportunity to sink deeply into your organism. The best first step is to fast: eat nothing, and drink only weak herbal tea, especially made of powdered ginger, until your wastes improve and your appetite intensifies. This is a general rule that like all other generalities has its exceptions, but these are rare. When your system shows signs of failing to digest properly you should almost always refraining from putting more food into your system until your digestive fire has revived.

WASHING

Washing your hands, feet, face, mouth, eyes and nose purifies your sense organs. First inspect your tongue for a thick, unpleasant-tasting coating. When present it shows that undigested or improperly digested food material has created a "coating" of poisonous ama in your digestive tract. A coating on your tongue may precede changes in the qualities of your wastes, so regular tongue inspection may enable you to interrupt indigestion before it can fully develop.

Scrape your tongue daily with a tongue scraper or a spoon made of silver, copper or stainless steel. Scrape your tongue back to front slowly five to ten times to express as much filth from its crypts as possible. Gargle salt water with a pinch of turmeric added occasionally to help keep your gums, mouth and throat healthy.

Brush your teeth daily, but lightly, to prevent damage to tooth enamel or gums. Millions of Indians still use twig toothbrushes, which are used once and then returned to Nature for recycling. Modern research has shown that toothbrushes may be one cause of recurrent infections since they can harbor colonies of pathogenic bacteria. Keep your toothbrush clean and dry at all times, and replace it frequently.

While twig toothbrushes floss your teeth as you brush, we in the West must use dental floss. Daily flossing is essential to dental health. So is daily use of

tooth powder or toothpaste, whose primary purpose is to invigorate and purify the gums. A sample tooth powder recipe:

> 5 parts alum or white oak bark powder
> 3 parts black pepper powder
> 2 parts rock salt (the black salt known as kala namak or the white
> salt known as saindhava is best)
> 1 part turmeric powder
> _ part natural camphor or clove oil

Clean your eyes with warm water that you have held in your mouth for a few
moments to absorb some of your saliva. Saliva is good for the eyes. Once a
week instill eye drops of honey, castor oil, rose water, or barberry or Triphala
tea, to expel excess Kapha. After cleaning out your nose with lightly salted water
instill a drop of oil into each nostril each day with the tip of your pinky. Drop
two or three drops of oil into each ear every week or two, to clean and lubricate them

MEDITATION

It is good to take a brief bath before meditating, but if this is inconvenient at
least wash your hands, feet and face thoroughly first. Meditating is one variety of eating, a consumption of subtle energies which the mind's subtle digestive fire will digest. Meditation, which appeases the hunger of the mind, is a
critical element of all daily programs. Insufficient or improper meditation keeps
the mind hungry, which makes it turn outward through its sense organs to
seek from sense objects, including especially physical food, that satisfaction
it should be finding within.

Using food to satisfy the mind alone without consideration for the body always
leads to disease. Good meditation nourishes your organism so well that your
body can learn to maintain itself on less food. Control of desire, which is the
mind's hunger, is the key to longevity and immortality.

Anything can be a meditation, as long as it is sincere and heartfelt. From the
strict viewpoint of your organism's health the simplest of all meditations involves
the sun, without whose heat and light we could not exist. Of all hues the gold-
en color of the sun is healthiest, most nourishing and most productive of strength
and vigor. Ayurveda advises daily ingestion of the gold color.

Yogis often gather this golden color by staring at the sun just as it comes over
the horizon each day for a few minutes, meditating on the solar magnificence
and munificence. You too can do this safely. Stare as long as you can, and once
the sun's brightness reaches a point of uncomfortable intensity close your eyes
and continue to stare for a few more moments through your closed eyelids.
Even a few minutes of sun gazing each day will invigorate your being and
improve your vision.

If you are wary of the sun or live in a cloudy climate you can obtain the gold
color by the Ayurvedic method of staring into a golden bowl filled with cow's
ghee, which is golden in color. Or you can use the procedure called trataka, in

which you place at arm's length at eye level a lamp containing ghee, which burns with a golden light, and stare fixedly into it until tears come. Or you can close your eyes and visualize the sun, or envision a glowing ball of hot gold. After any of these procedures wash your eyes, and put a drop or two of pure rose water into each if any excess heat seem to remain.

MASSAGE

Touch is the skin's sense. Remember that the skin and the digestive tract are the physical barriers that separate you from your environment. They control entrance into your system, permitting nutrients access while refusing entry to pathogens. Bodily wastes can also be excreted through both the skin and the gut. When excretion through other channels becomes inefficient, or when wastes pile up past the capacity of the excretory organs to deal with them, the excess waste is directed out through the skin. Skin disease usually develops when the skin is clogged with toxic wastes. The health of the skin is thus intimately connected with the health of the digestive tract. Skin disease improves when digestive function improves, and when the skin is cleansed of all its impurities and toned to vibrancy the digestive tract also becomes healthier.

Every human being needs regular oil massage. While self-massage is adequate for most people most of the time, everyone should seek professional massage from time to time. Massage makes the skin soft and unctuous and controls Vata by reducing Vata's cold, dry, light, rough and erratic qualities. Its rhythmic motion allays joint and muscle stiffness and makes all body movements free and rhythmic. Massage increases the circulation of the blood, encouraging quicker removal of metabolic wastes. Massage also relaxes the body prior to more vigorous exercise.

V people require massage more than do P and K types because the sense of touch is most acute in V people, so acute that touch can sometimes be painful. Touch can also be therapeutic. V people need to be touched more than do others because touch helps ground them in a level of consciousness appropriate for living in the world. Massage provides therapeutic touch and softens the acuteness of the sense of touch.

V people are also more prone to damage by radiation than are other types, and research has shown that vegetable oil in the diet and applied to the skin helps protect individuals from the destructive effects of radiation. The internal and external use of medicated oils is Ayurveda's fundamental strategy for balancing V people and managing Vata-caused conditions.

To protect their health and sanity all V people should visit a competent masseur or masseuse regularly, once a week if possible but not less than once a month. Routinely scheduling the massage for the same weekday each time at the same time of day will reinforce and enhance the massage's effects.

P individuals should go for variety in massage, sampling shiatsu, accupressure, polarity and various other techniques to keep their minds occupied. P tissues are inherently tender and irritable and need careful manipulation to avoid aggravation.

K types require firm hands, deeply penetrating fingers, and a technique bordering on harshness to awaken the sluggish circulation and eliminate cellular wastes. They should use oil sparingly or dispense with it altogether. People of dual constitutions should select massage based on the season of the year and their own individual conditions.

It is good to use oil from a plant that grows or could grow in your area. You should select the oil according to season (using heating oils like mustard or sesame in the winter and cooling oils like coconut or olive in the summer), climate (wet oils like sesame and castor in dry climates and drying oils like safflower in a wet climate), and individual constitution. Sandalwood oil is probably the best of all medicinal oils; it reduces the Pitta and Kapha-causing properties of any oils it may be mixed with as it promotes mental balance and coolness.

All oils are good for V people, but sesame, almond, mustard and castor are usually best. Olive oil, cocoa butter and coconut oil are optimal for Ps, with some fragrant oil like lavender or sandalwood added. Ks should avoid oil and concentrate on dry massage, but for skin lubrication they can apply sunflower, safflower or, in winter, mustard oils. VP people need less oil than do pure Vs but can use most oils and should get regular massages. PKs should usually use sunflower or corn oil, and VKs can use mustard, almond, sunflower or corn as they please. VKs should get frequent massages.

For general body massage you can mix an ounce (30 ml) of an aromatic oil like sandalwood with a quart (1 liter) of an oil appropriate for current conditions. V, VP and VK types with poor circulation to the extremities may choose to add in one to two teaspoons (5 to 10 ml) of oil of wintergreen or eucalyptus oil per quart of their main oil. Pine needle oil helps combat tendencies to muscle spasm, and pure jasmine oil (as much as one ounce per pint) can be used for an aphrodisiac effect. Unmedicated vegetable oils except castor oil should never be applied to rheumatic joints. Castor oil can be applied to any part of the skin at any time. A little oil of garlic in the castor oil to act as a counter-irritant helps the rheumatic part cleanse itself.

Given that the skin eats oil as surely as if you had put it into your mouth you should never apply to your body mineral oil, or any vegetable oil that has been perfumed or colored with chemicals. You can store your massage oil in the refrigerator, but avoid preserving it for longer than three months. If you store your oil in a red bottle and expose it to the sun daily for forty days its essential heat will increase, which will improve its efficiency in Vata and Vata-Kapha conditions like body aches and pains. Storing oil in a blue bottle and exposing it to the sun daily for forty days makes it cooler, which will enhance its effects on prickly heat, burns, and other high-heat Pitta conditions.

Follow the flow of body energy when you massage yourself to avoid diverting Vata from its normal direction. You can do this by working in the direction that your hairs grow. Work from your hands and feet towards your trunk, and from outwards inward. Apply a little extra oil over your body's vital parts—heart, navel, genitals, joints, anus, and any as yet unoiled sense organs—and apply it liberally over all hairy areas, like your head, armpits, pubes, and chest.

Your hair's nutrition is linked with the nutrition of the bones, and oil on your head hair also helps control the Vata in your mind. Once a week work some oil into your scalp and wait twenty minutes or so for it to soak in before you wash it out. Oil massage of the head relaxes both brain and body and strengthens the sense organs.

When you have no time to massage your whole body at least massage the soles of your feet. Oil massage of the feet promotes sound sleep. If your eyes are weak oil both your great toenails nightly. Avoid massage when your digestive tract is full of ama. Abnormal bodily wastes and a heavily coated tongue indicate ama even if there are no other symptoms, but most acute diseases, especially fevers, are associated with extensive ama.

EXERCISE

Exercise may be passive like massage, active like aerobics, or both passive and active like Hatha Yoga. Exercise increases the body's stamina and resistance to disease by facilitating the action of the immune system. It clears all channels, promotes circulation and waste disposal, and destroys fat. Regular exercise even reduces anxiety and produces a sense of well-being by stimulating the release of endorphins and enkephalins, which helps explain why exercise can be addictive.

V people become addicted to vigorous exercise because it temporarily exhausts them, preventing them from thinking at their normal hyperspeed rate, and because exercise temporarily increases their pain threshold. Pain reduction is important to the normally pain-sensitive V person. Excessive vigorous exercise exhausts the body, however, which disturbs Vata. Also, the dullness of mind which vigorous exercise engenders is only temporary. The rebound effect makes the mind work even more vigorously and chaotically afterwards, as if to make up for lost time.

Many V people are attracted to running or jogging, practices that put great pressure on their inherently weak joints. Joint injuries in V people are more likely to become complicated or to result in arthritis than similar injuries in other types. Some Vs are attracted to sports like handball, which require the intense bursts of energy that Vs have in abundance. V people who do invest in such overactivity, however, eventually experience total energy wipeout. Mild, regular exercise like Yoga, Tai Chi or walking is always better for V people than is intense exertion. Contemplative exercises like Yoga and Tai Chi are especially good for V types because they promote mental equanimity.

Vs tend to be fidgety anyway, and the energy that a confirmed fidgeter burns off in a day is equivalent to that expended in jogging several miles. Rhythmic exercise is always better for V types than are chaotic workouts. For example, regular weight training with light weights is far better for V types than is sporadic aerobic exhaustion. V people who are addicted to jogging and running may find an alternative in a rebounder. Participatory exercise like folk dancing may also satisfy their requirements for motion.

Since V people hate routines and love to try new things they should feel free to begin with any sort of exercise they please. Once they have created an exercise habit they should then tone down the vigor and enhance the stabilization. External sources of heat like steam baths and hot tubs further stimulate their circulation. VP people require less heat than do pure Vs but should generally observe V-type exercise guidelines.

P people love vigorous exercise like weightlifting because it feeds their aggressiveness and makes them all the more intense, irritable and driven. Competitive sports like tennis excite them because they are naturally competitive and love the thrill of competition. An optimal exercise for a P person provides this competitiveness without permitting it to reinforce the natural P egotism. Team sports like basketball and volleyball which emphasize cooperation and downplay individual heroics, or sports like backpacking which permit you to compete against yourself, are best for P types. Tai Chi and Yoga can be good for Ps if they use them to cool their fire and balance their aggression.

Ps should indulge in external sources of heat with care. If Nature had meant Ps to lie for hours in the sun She would have given them dark skins. Ps should use a sun blocking lotion with this in mind, and should go under cover when they begin to get too warm. Swimming is great for Ps because it is cooling; it helps reduce fire, as do water skiing and snow skiing. Swimming is an excellent, simple form of exercise that is especially good for Vs and Ps but is suitable for everyone.

K people really *need* vigorous exercise. Many K people need strenuous encouragement to develop an exercise habit, but once it develops the K person will normally stick with it. Ks usually do not like to have to involve themselves intensively with the activity and so tend to choose exercises like bicycling which can be done on autopilot. Such repetitive activities reinforce the repetitive, habitual nature of the K organism, however. Strenuous sports, or complicated aerobic routines, are better. Yoga and Tai Chi can be good if they are used to stimulate and energize the organism.

K and PK types alone should indulge in activities that strain the physical organism to its limits, like ice hockey or lumberjacking. Most VKs do not have the same inherent stamina because of the influence of Vata. They require vigorous exercise regularly but not continuously, and need liberal doses of heat. Though Ks should avoid repetitive exercise those who need to be motivated to exercise can begin with repetitive activities, like long-distance running or calisthenics. Complexity can then be gradually added into the program.

Exercise cannot benefit you if you exhaust yourself with it. Ayurveda's rule is never to exert more than half your capacity at any one time. If you know you will be exhausted after, say, one hour of bicycling you should not cycle more than half an hour at a time until your stamina improves. In extreme climates your energy will be dissipated faster, and you should not exercise even to half your capacity. Do not exercise when you are ill with respiratory diseases, such as chronic cough or cold, or when you have any severe inflammation or severe indigestion. Children should not begin strenuous exercise too early in life, nor should strenuous exercise be continued too long into old age.

Wrongful exercise can put body parts out of balance with one another, overemphasizing one area while neglecting others. Even appropriate exercise can have undesirable effects when overdone. Vigorous exercise increases the need for physical food to replace the nutrients burned to supply energy. This extra food requires extra energy for digestion, and since this energy must be obtained at the mind's expense overexercising will dull the mind. Ayurveda always encourages meditative exercise, like Yoga and Tai Chi, to prevent this mental dullness and to ensure proper energy flow throughout the organism. Such practices regularize V people, calm P people, invigorate K people, and help integrate those with dual constitutions.

Ayurveda also suggests that exercise be performed with rhythmic breathing. Breathing expels gaseous wastes from the body and welcomes Prana, the life force, in. Good breathing purifies the lungs; poor breathing makes the lungs unhealthy and disturbs the colon and the bones. To make your exercise effective your breath must flow regularly, evenly and deeply.

The simplest breathing exercise you can do is to sit and concentrate on breathing from deep in your abdomen, slowing the flow gradually and effortlessly until you are taking only a few breaths each minute.

Yogis say that each individual is born with a specified number of breaths available to them, and that as soon as these breaths are used up the individual dies. The faster you breathe the sooner you will use up your breaths, and the shorter your life will be. You live longer by breathing slower, which is another argument against excessive vigorous aerobic exercise. Whatever your exercise or meditation you should concentrate on your breathing for a few minutes each day, sitting with your back straight and breathing with your abdomen instead of your chest.

My teacher Vimalananda used to say that even if you ignore all other rules of routine you can still maintain good health as long as you:

Keep *your bowels moving* (keep your colon clean)

Keep *your body moving* (exercise regularly)

Keep *your breath moving* (always breathe slowly and deeply).

It is better to take the time every day to make sure that your colon empties properly than to perform stringent Ayurvedic or Yogic purifications for a few weeks at a time and then ignore your bowels for the rest of the year. It is better to take a few minutes each day to move your body, even if only by walking around the block or performing isometric exercises in your bedroom, than to run long-distance races once or twice a year and lie around like a sloth in between them. It is better to spend five minutes each day breathing quietly, deeply, and slowly, regenerating your stores of Prana, than it is to perform fancy Pranayamas (yogic breathing exercises) on special occasions and ignore your breathing otherwise.

The crest jewel of exercises is the Sun Salutation (*Surya Namaskara*), a sequence of Yogic postures performed with rhythmic breathing. Each posture has associated with it a *mantra*, a specialized sound pattern which invigorates the subtle body as the posture invigorates the physical body. The breathing helps tie the two bodies together. The Sun Salutation is balancing and harmonizing even if you do not know the mantras, however, because it helps to integrate all the various identities (spiritual, mental and physical) into one. It is simultaneously a meditation and an exercise.

The Sun Salutation appears deceptively simple. Begin with one to three rounds daily and work slowly up to a dozen or more. V people should perform Sun Salutations slowly and meditatively, K people quickly and vigorously, and P people at a medium pace. P people especially should strive to learn the appropriate mantras for each movement, to help engage their active powers of focus.

The Sun Salute - Surya Namaskara

Stand quietly with your palms together and inhale and exhale slowly.

Brings your palms apart as you inhale slowly, stretching your arms and head back. With your arms open and your palms facing upwards, arch easily backwards.

Exhale slowly, keeping your head between your arms and slowly bend forward from your waist. Keeping your knees straight as you go down relax your head, neck, shoulders and arms. Touch the floor with your hands if you can.

Bending both knees place your palms flat on either side of your feet. Stretch your left leg back keeping your left knee and toe on the floor. Inhale slowly as you stretch your chin upwards.

Bring your feet parallel to each other and raise your hips up into a jack-knife position, forming a triangle with your chin locked to your chest. Retain the breath.

Move your feet back and lower yourself until your toes, knees, chest and forehead—but not your abdomen—are touching the floor. Exhale slowly as you lower yourself.

Inhale slowly as you easily arch back your spine with your chin up, hips and toes on the floor and elbows slightly bent.

Exhale slowly as you raise your hips into a jack-knife position, again forming a triangle. Keep your heels to the floor with your chin locked on your chest.

Inhale slowly as your bring your left leg up between both hands. Keep your right knee on the floor and your palms flat with your chin up.

Exhale slowly as you bring both feet together, knees straight, bending forward from the hips. Relax your neck, head, and arms.

Slowly raise up, inhaling as you stretch your hands outwards and then upwards, arching back your arms and head with the palms upward.

Exhale slowly while bringing your palms together and closing your eyes.

Then repeat the entire sequence, but this time move your right leg back prior to the jack-knife position, and bring it forward first when coming out of the second jack-knife.

Exhale slowly while bringing your palms together and closing your eyes.

Carefully observe the different changes in your body: the increase of your heat, your breath, your heart beat.

Hold each of the twelve postures for three seconds at first. Once you become familiar with the Sun Salute each posture will flow smoothly one into the other. Allow your breath to flow freely as your body shifts from pose to pose, avoiding any feeling of breathlessness. Above all go slowly, according to your own to your own capacity. If you have a history of high blood pressure or heart trouble please check with your physician before you do this exercise.

The Sun Salutation is the supreme exercise because it balances and activates the body, controls and conditions the mind, and also possesses a spiritual aspect. It is a salute to the sun, the source of our life. Even if you cannot work the Sun Salutation into your daily routine no V is so disorganized, no P so busy and no K so indolent that they cannot do some kind of exercise. At the very least you can walk, an exercise which tones the bowels, relaxes the body and promotes digestion, all the while preserving mental clarity. If all else fails you can laugh. Laughter burns calories, improves lung function, oxygenates the blood, invites Prana into the system, releases endorphins, and strengthens the immune system. And it is so easy to do!

BATHING

Ayurveda advocates the warm water bath; Yoga advises the use of cold water. The body cools minutes after exposure to hot water as the blood vessels that dilated with heat contract in reaction. A cold shower has the opposite effect, making you warm within a few minutes as the vessels constricted by the cold dilate.

A good compromise for V people, who require heat, is to luxuriate in a warm bath or shower and then, after imbibing enough heat to feel warm, to preserve that warmth by rinsing with cold water at the end. P people should if possible adapt themselves to cool (but not cold) showers and baths, to help remove their excess heat. K types should adapt to cool water, to invigorate themselves. No one should bathe for at least an hour after eating, to avoid drawing blood away from the gut where it is required for digestion. Avoid bathing temporarily in case of diarrhea, distention, chronic cold or indigestion, and in most acute diseases in which ama predominates.

Intensely hot water applied directly to the head drains strength from the sense organs. While you can use shampoo regularly for the hair and scalp you should soap your body only in case of real grime. Soap robs the skin of its protective mantle and encourages growth of the bacteria which cause body odor. Soap is especially bad for mucus membranes (anus, genitals, nipples, etc.). Instead of soap use clay or barley or chickpea flour to soak up the oil left after the massage and the sweat left after the exercise. Flour draws out the wastes excreted by the system after massage and exercise and tones the skin without drying it or leaving a soap film. Soap should never be used on most skin diseases.

If you have not applied oil to your whole body you can incorporate oil into a skin paste. Mix half a cup of oil with a cup of chickpea, barley or even wheat flour, and add one-quarter to one-half teaspoon of turmeric powder to assist in skin purification. Add just enough water to make it a thick but spreadable paste and apply it evenly, rubbing it in as you apply. If possible let it dry until it begins to crack. This acts as a mask, or pack, for the whole body.

A mental bath should always accompany the physical bath, to awaken the mind and enkindle its digestive fires. Specific bathing mantras do exist, but any devotional song or hymns, or in fact any song or chant which you enjoy, will help satisfy your mind and will make for a more satisfying bath.

Lifestyle

It is good to perform your routine in the morning before you go out into the world, since it applies "armor" to you for your foray into the external environment. Failure to properly shield yourself against the dangers of the outside world opens you to invasion by destabilizing outside forces, be they humans or bacteria. This is not the sort of "armor" that insulates you from beneficial energies; it merely allows you to screen incoming influences to decide which you would like to take. By selecting beneficial experiences and shielding yourself against divisive forces you can create for yourself an internal environment which will be conducive to your total health, according to your own personal constitution.

CLOTHING

Your clothes are the removable part of your external armor. Clothes are more important than ever today, given the preponderance of evil influences circulating in society. Your clothing should always be light and airy, made of natural fibers like cotton, wool or linen. Silk is the fabric which best insulates against adverse external influences too subtle to be otherwise avoided. This is why Indian priests like to use silk clothing during ritual worship. Some experts maintain that rayon also possesses this property.

Always wear clean clothes, and never wear clothing, flowers or footwear that anyone else has worn, since these items too easily pick up an individual's innate personality vibrations. No one's vibration is better for you than your own except that of a saint, someone who has reached a higher level of integration than you have. Use of a saint's clothing, flowers or footwear actually helps harmonize your being.

In India people lovingly worship both the feet and the footwear of their saints. They know that energy is brought into the body through the crown of the head and exits through the soles of the feet. The energy which exits from you will be polluted and miasmic if you are unhealthy mentally or physically, or it will be tonic and healthful if you are well-balanced and integrated, as saints are. Applying henna leaf paste or rubbing ghee with a small bronze bowl on the soles of the feet can reduce fever by extracting abnormal heat from the system.

Your footwear absorbs much of the energy that your feet emit. Footwear is not allowed in the house in India or other Oriental countries because no matter how clean it is externally it still traps some of this polluted energy. Footwear pollutes whatever it comes in contact with as surely as muddy shoes track up a clean floor. Since your own use of your own footwear will to some extent affect your consciousness adversely you will do well to go barefoot whenever possible, especially inside the house. Another reason to go barefoot is shoe leather itself, which being the skin of a dead animal tends to pollute one's consciousness. Shoes made out of rubber are an improvement, but they are said to adversely affect the eyes. Strict Indian Yogis always either go barefoot or wear wooden sandals.

EMPLOYMENT

Work consumes at least a third of our lives. Success or failure at your chosen profession affects your self-confidence, your self-worth and the self-validity of your personality. Your work should agree with your prakriti.

V people love to work at jobs that require sudden bursts of intense energy, because they naturally work that way. Such work exhausts them, however, and should be avoided. Even though they despise and resist anything boring, repetitive or routine, ideal employment for a V is somewhat repetitive, to discipline the normally erratic V nature. V people should avoid places where the air is exceptionally cool and dry, such as the clean room of an electronics-manufacturing outfit, or exceptionally dusty, like a feed or fertilizer mill, even though such work would have the benefit of being routine.

Vs need a soothing home and work environment to smooth out their rough edges. They need adequate rest, and should if possible arrange for a 10-minute catnap during the afternoon, the Vata time of day. Vs should not schedule important meetings for late afternoon unless they want to sleep or sail through them. V people must pace themselves carefully and resist the temptation to try to do everything at once. It is sometimes acutely painful for V people to be steady or endure tedium, but it is essential for them to do so.

V types are excellent original thinkers, and if they theorize for a living they must be sure to keep themselves grounded with a fixed routine of massage, exercise, sleep and food. This also applies to those Vs who because of their love of frequent change are led into travel-related professions, like the airlines. Any V person who wishes to enjoy the constant stimulation of such a job, the continual excitement of seeing new places and meeting new people, must observe strict control over all other aspects of his or her life. Change and excitement are intoxicants for V people, and like all other intoxicants they are meant for occasional indulgence only. The challenge is to find a job that has sufficient excitement to hold a V's interest but is sufficiently routine to prevent imbalances.

P people are practical to a fault. They take ideas dreamed up by V theoreticians and apply them to real situations. Ps are realists and enjoy the palpabilities of reality; for example, they tend to be obsessed with numbers and time, like how many new accounts can be obtained per month, or how many appointments can be squeezed into one eight-hour day. Ps are by nature aggressive and self-promoting. To them everything is a contest, and all contests deserve to be won. They must be in the forefront of all activity, first across the finish line in any competition. They invite as many stimuli into their lives as they can cram in, and demand perfect functioning from their bodies at all times.

Ideal employment for Ps would include sufficient challenge to keep them occupied without the stress of severe competition. Teaching, for example, provides a P with the intellectual challenge of communicating his or her knowledge to others without needing to lead into the perpetual comparison with others in the same profession that a career in sales might. Ps ought also to avoid physically irritating work situations, like welding or metal casting which involve intense heat that might increase Pitta. Violence of any kind is not good for Ps, even in the movies.

P people who do choose stimulating employment always struggle against irritability and impatience. Ps love to plan and become enthusiastic about their plans; they do not take obstacles or delays well. They need to be willing to listen to other people and refrain from dismissing others' ideas out of hand. At mid-day, the Pitta time of day, Ps become exceptionally hungry and irritable and should avoid confrontations before they are able to eat. Ps find it hard to separate their professions from their private lives. No one should take their work home with them, but P people must be stricter than others need be in this separation of career and family. They need to set aside time to "burn," to make themselves available to their families for seemingly non-essential pursuits.

Ks are not known as either original thinkers or outstanding engineers, but a good K makes a great administrator. The innate K stability and balance makes any business they are associated run as if on "greased wheels." A K whose position is almost totally routine and repetitive must consciously inject change and stimulation into his or her life. Even if it only involves rearranging furniture in office or home, any effort to make frequent changes in their physical environment is therapeutic for K types. Ks should also ensure that if their work is not physically active their leisure time is. Competition is good for them, though they may find it stressful, and they should avoid accepting neat, tidy answers to complex problems, even in unimportant matters.

Morning is the Kapha time of day, and Ks should not expect to be able to do much creative work then. They should keep the mornings for routine work, which Ks can do better than anyone else, and tackle thornier questions around mid-day or in the afternoon when the cosmos provides them Pitta for decision-making power and Vata to encourage speculation, respectively. Making your constitution work for you, not against you, in every aspect of your life is one of life's great challenges.

PETS

Pets are extensions of their owners' personalities, small versions of their masters. Most people prefer pets with whom they can innately relate, who reflect their own character traits. It is better though to keep a pet who is therapeutic for your own imbalances. V people do well with dogs, for example, for a canine's lovable, sloppy, openheartedness warms, reassures, relaxes and stabilizes the Vs cold, fearful, fickle nature. K individuals do better with small animals like birds. An avian's light, bright cheerfulness helps offset some of a Ks natural ponderousness, sluggishness and fixity.

Some K people find large dogs beneficial in that both dog and owner need vigorous exercise, and responsibility for the canine encourages the K person to exercise along with the dog. Some V types do well with small furry high-strung animals like guinea pigs and hamsters that elicit maternal instinct from their owners.

P personalities are sometimes too overbearing to obtain much incentive for self-development from the simpler personalities of birds and beasts. Ps should not take the easy way out and select an animal who is too easy to get along with, nor one who is so aggressive that the two beings feed off one another's instincts to violence. A large long-lived bird like a parrot may be complex enough to demand attention from a P. Cats, who have strongly-held opinions about most subjects including their masters, present continuous challenges to the probing P mind and make perhaps the best P pets. The P has to keep up with the feline, and this is a refreshingly new experience for many hotshot Ps.

SPOUSE

Just as you would not throw out a pet who did not perfectly meet your needs you should not discard a spouse who is not a perfect match for you. But you will be benefited if you know something of your constitution before you select either a pet or a spouse.

Ancient Indian sexology insists that individuals of like constitution be paired together—Vs with Vs, Ps with Ps, and Ks with Ks—because of their inherent sexual proclivities. For example, Ks are not particularly oversexed but do become quite lusty once their natural indolence is conquered. Because of their innate physical strength two Ks will not easily wear each other out with their persistent readiness for intercourse. Two V partners excite each other easily and become easily exhausted, which is fine, since there is a sense of mutuality present. A V and a K paired together might experience mutual frustration: first the V would feel lack of interest from the partner, then after days or weeks when the Ks sexual appetite was awakened and became ravenous the V might be too worn out to respond with equal ardor.

Ayurvedic wisdom adds that like types make better mates because of similar mental processes and attitudes. For example, V people generally cannot hold onto money. They tend to fritter it away, spend it on impulse, or donate it to some "cause." P people calculate well, plan, and save and spend with conscious design. A pure P and a pure V married to one another would probably tear out their mutual hair over the partner's fiscal habits.

Unfortunately, two people of like dispositions are likely to have like defects. Two V people living together will tend to feed off one another's chaotic energies and will often end up bouncing off the walls, babbling at one another in blue streaks without much communication. Two K people could conceivably so immobilize each other that they could live together for years with little interaction. Two P people will rarely be able to resist competing against one another, trying to gain the upper hand in the relationship. Their habitual mutual irritation can lead to great and terrible tussles interspersed with periods of uneasy truce.

Prakriti is the problem. Recall that Kapha is the force which forces Water and Earth to cooperate together, even though they would prefer to ignore one another. At the core of their beings K people feel a desire to avoid confrontation and no effort from within or without can completely overcome that tendency. Even if a lone K can exert sufficient will force to encourage self-transformation it is too easy for two Ks living together to persist in old habits and reinforce each other's innate tendencies.

Likewise, heat is not the only reason for a Ps inborn antagonism. Pitta's job is to balance two mutually antagonistic elements: Fire and Water. Two P people living together are almost certain to project competition at one another; it comes naturally. Two Vs in the same household are unlikely ever to develop the discipline they so urgently need. Vata has to try to impose limitation on Air, which resists all limitation, with the help of Ether, which can exert only an ethereal influence. Two people of like prakriti always tend to reinforce one another's constitutional weaknesses.

Ps can give Vs organization for their mental chaos, and Vs can give Ps continuous communication challenges. But if there is imbalance the V wind will blow like a bellows on the P fire and incinerate the relationship, or the P fire will heat up the V air and expand it like a balloon until it flies off or bursts. Vs can get stability and balance from Ks, and shake them out of their ponderousness in return. If not their mutual coldness will cause the V air to solidify K into stubbornness, or the K stickiness to obstruct Vs free flow. Ps heat up and activate Ks; Ks cool and ballast Ps. If the P is too hot, though, the K will boil over, and if the K is too wet the P will get drowned.

Two people who live together long enough begin to rub off on one another, and even begin to look like one another. Any two people who sleep next to one another nightly enter each other's aura, even if there is no sexual relationship between them, because of the proximity and the lowering of defenses which occurs during sleep. Proximity may in some cases be enough to promote integration, if the couple involved is committed to the relationship, but the force of Nature is often too strong to overcome with good intentions alone. For example, a V-K match is unlikely to succeed without a significant area of shared interest, like a job or a hobby, to provide the personality welding which is needed to make a marriage a success but which their relationship lacks since they both lack ample Fire.

The whole issue becomes much murkier when the VP, PK and VK permutations are added to the picture. A VP mated with a PK form one of the most stable of relationships; both have enough Fire energy to communicate with one another, and the V of the one balances the K of the other. A VK and a PK can form a good match, though their shared K stubbornness will tend to amplify the differences between them. A VK and a VP may make a good spiritual pair, but the stability of their mundane life will be reduced because of the shared V influence.

Your choice must fundamentally depend on your ambitions for relationship in this lifetime. If you want a stable relationship with a compatible spouse, select someone of your own constitutional type. The mutual excess that occurs in such pairings is easier to endure than the strained dynamic inherent in a pairing of two people whose constitutions differ radically. Two constitutionally similar individuals involved with one another intuitively understand the forces that motivate their partners, because those same forces motivate them. If you do not want to have to put a lot of energy into a relationship, look for a spouse who is of your metabolic type.

If you wish to use a relationship as a vehicle for self-evolution, select a partner who will stimulate you and shake you up, who will offer you what you lack and to whom you can provide complementary energy. Be warned, though, that such a course may find you and your spouse eating, drinking and being merry in widely differing ways as a result of your constitutional variance.

SURROUNDINGS

The above rules hold for all interpersonal interactions. You should also evaluate potential friends and comrades according to how harmonizing their influence will be. Friendship with self-destructive individuals will magnify any self-destructiveness you have not yet expunged from your being; camaraderie with the empathetic will increase your own empathy. When you choose to associate with negative individuals you will pick up physical, mental and spiritual defects from them; this is Sanga Dosha. Satsanga, which is association with strong, healthy, spiritual people, allows their harmoniousness to rub off on you.

Physical and mental characteristics should also influence your choice of residence. Pure V people do best in hot, humid climates like Hawaii and the Gulf Coast, and find frigid climates almost unbearable. Pure K people require hot, arid climates like the Western desert to balance themselves, and pure P types shun torrid climates and adore the cold. V and K people both need regular exposure to the sun (while carefully avoiding overexposure!). Ps must be particularly wary of the sun.

Socially and culturally you might choose to make your home in as opulent a neighborhood as possible, with neighbors of like minds and like tastes, and avoid any contact with poverty to prevent your sensibilities from being disturbed by unsettling sights. This attitude would maximize your ability to manifest your own physical wealth, and would enhance your Earth and Water energies.

You might, if you chose to maximize your spiritual nature, live in a simple and limited style in a simple dwelling with simple friends as neighbors, avoiding the company of the rich and powerful whose minds are immersed in the mire of the world. This would enhance the Air and Ether energies in your organism.

And if you want to exercise your mental faculties you could adapt yourself to whatever environment you found yourself in, experiencing people of all sorts and styles, maintaining under all circumstances perfect presence of mind. This would strengthen your Fire energy.

Varied vegetables cook together into a stew, each offering part of its own individuality, each accepting part of the identity of the others. Just as you have a responsibility to yourself to eat healthily and to live healthily you have the responsibility of choosing healthy associates, healthy environments, and healthy pastimes. This is why Ayurveda insists that all your spare time should be spent with your "elders." An elder is anyone who is older than you are in maturity and experience; chronological age is irrelevant. The society which has no elders must be shunned, no matter how advanced materially or artistically it may be.

SLEEP

Ayurveda calls sleep the "Wet-nurse of the World," for sleep nourishes beings with motherliness and promotes their growth. Sleep's essence is inertia, bodily inertia with mental relaxation; it is closely associated with Kapha.

Night is the time for sleep, after the personality tires of projecting itself externally. Ten-minute daily catnaps are good for V types. Long naps are permitted for anyone in the peak of summer, when days are hot and nights are short. Otherwise sleeping during the day increases Kapha. Only the very young, the very old, the very weak and those exhausted by sex, intoxicants, disease, travel, overwork or other physical or emotional trauma should nap longer than ten or fifteen minutes in an afternoon. Sometimes a nap before eating will benefit a case of acute indigestion but usually, unless you have been awake all night, sleeping during the day will produce ama.

Early to bed and early to rise is ideal for everyone. Evening is the Kapha time of night, the time when it is natural to wind down and prepare for repose. Staying up after midnight aggravates both Pitta and Vata. Midnight is the Pitta time of night, and Ps especially should not be awake then, lest their appetites balloon and they be tempted to eat. Ps sometimes wake up in the middle of the night hungry or, if they have ulcers, in pain from the acid Pitta has caused the body to secrete then. Vata discourages sound sleep during the hours that it governs just before dawn. V people in particular need to go to bed early, to enable Kapha to promote sound sleep until Vata arouses them.

No one should consume a full physical or mental meal less than two hours before bed. All physical and mental digestive processes should be complete before surrendering to sleep. Meditation and nervine herbs like valerian are permissible for pre-sleep consumption. V people often find a cup of warm milk with a pinch of saffron in it to be soporific.

Sitting up provides the most alert sleep and is the best sleeping position. Sleeping on your right side is most relaxing, and on your left, most promotive of digestion. Sleeping on your back disturbs Vata, and habitually sleeping on your stomach disturbs everything. Yogis who do not sleep sitting up prefer to sleep on their right sides, to encourage the function of their left nostrils. This cools and relaxes the body and makes it easier to control, which is essential for Yoga.

Individuals who wish to amply enjoy the pleasures of the world should sleep on their left sides, to promote functioning of their right nostrils. The right nostril heats and activates the body and increases the organism's interest in food, sleep and sex. This assists you to better externalize your personality, to enable it to better enjoy sensuousness.

Sleeping on the back allows both nostrils to function together, which discourages body-mind-spirit integration and indirectly promotes disease by encouraging energy to leave the body. Sleeping on the stomach promotes disease directly by obstructing deep, healthy breathing.

To lie with the crown of your head into the east and your feet into the west promotes meditative sleep. Sleeping with your head into the north draws energy out of the body, disturbing body-mind-spirit integration. This is good for astral travel, but not for health. If you sleep with your head into the south energy will be drawn into your body, improving your health. Head into the west promotes disturbing dreams.

Before sleep always wash your hands, feet and face, massage your feet with a little oil, and meditate for a few moments, to allow the day's negativity to dissipate before you enter into the arms of slumber. If you have trouble with frequent wet dreams you can wash your legs and feet in cold water before retiring to draw energy away from the genitals and reduce the likelihood of nocturnal emission.

You should never go to bed to read, write or think, and you should arise immediately on waking. Never sleep in a kitchen or any other place where food is prepared, since both the savory odors and the subtle vibrations in the area will alert your digestive tract and disturb your sleep.

The ideal form of sleep is called Yoga Nidra, a state of complete physical inertness with retention of mental alertness and awareness. The more perfectly you can approach this ideal, the better prepared your organism will be for its new incarnation at dawn, when your routine begins again.

Chapter Six
Balance

Structure in life helps reduce the effects of stress. Stress, or rather improper reaction to stress, creates new diseases and worsens pre-existent ones. Stress permits alien beings like viruses and cancerous cells to colonize new territory by impairing the immune system's ability to respond to invasion.

Stress occurs every time you have to adapt to a new situation. Every time your surroundings—your physical, mental, emotional, social and spiritual circumstances—change you must change along with them, and develop a new equilibrium. Your immunity is your resilience, your capacity to roll with the punches and snap back to normal after even the lowest of blows. As stress increases, strain on the immune system grows, and when the strain becomes too great your immune protection fails and you develop an illness.

Stress seems to be proliferating; even unborn children today sometimes develop peptic ulcers. No one is immune from exposure to all stress, but we can improve our immunity to the stresses we do encounter. Whatever the variety and the timing of your stress, your natural reaction to it will be determined by your constitution. You will react as your genes instruct you to react unless you have conditioned your body to react differently. Specific patterns of Vata-Pitta-Kapha derangement must develop in order for specific diseases to manifest, but all patterns of derangement are fundamentally due to the weakness of your immunity, which is your individuality.

Prana, Tejas and Ojas

Prana is the life force, equivalent to the chi or ki in Oriental medicine. It strings body, mind and spirit together on a single strand of breath, like pearls on a thread, and causes them to live, to act together as a single organism. Tejas is the force of transmutation, which permits body, mind and spirit to influence one another in spite of their different planes of existence. Ojas, the subtlest manifestation of the force of immunity, is the glue that cements these pieces together and integrates your being. Prana, Tejas and Ojas unite body, mind and spirit.

Vata, Pitta and Kapha, the Three Doshas, are the gross manifestations of Prana, Tejas and Ojas, which are not doshas at all. Vata is the more unstable form of Prana, Pitta the more reactive form of Tejas, and Kapha the more inert form of Ojas. When physical, mental and spiritual digestion are at their peak Vata, Pitta and Kapha are produced from Prana, Tejas and Ojas in quantities just sufficient to perform necessary bodily functions. Poor digestion allows greater production of these reactive by-products, reducing thereby the amount of the essential forces that the organism has available to it. Increased Vata, Pitta and Kapha production also requires increased excretion, and further energy loss.

We obtain Prana from our atmosphere and from our food. Breathing recharges Prana immediately. Prana is not oxygen, any more than Kapha is mucus or Pitta is bile. Prana is the life force; oxygen is one of its carrier substances. Food and water also carry Prana. While most of our nutrients are absorbed into the circulation from the small intestine, Prana is absorbed from the colon. Modern research shows that substances called volatile fatty acids are absorbed from the colon into the circulation and can act as a significant energy source for the system. These volatile fatty acids, like oxygen, are carriers of Prana. The health of our lungs and colons determines how much Prana we can absorb, and thus how alive we feel.

When the lungs or the large intestine function inefficiently our bodies absorb Prana inefficiently and Vata is generated in increased amounts. Vata and Prana are alike, both being airy, intense, expansive and subtle, but Vata is not inherently balancing and nutritive, as Prana is. Unless Vata is regularly excreted from the system it causes disease. Although disturbed Vata can affect any dhatu it shows special affinity for Bone. The health of Bone is thus intimately tied to the health of the lungs and the colon. Hence Vimalananda's advice to keep the body (the bones) moving, the bowels (the colon) moving, and the breath (the lungs) moving.

Pathologies in the lungs, bones and large intestine are often related. For example, women who smoke lose more calcium from their bones because of the effect of carbon monoxide in the smoke on blood chemistry. Likewise, balancing one of these organs can benefit the others. Dry ginger mixed with jaggery (solidified sugar cane juice) improves the flow of urine and feces and, when it is given to patients of upper respiratory congestion, may relieve this congestion by relieving congestion in the colon. Sometimes medicated enemas are administered to control an attack of asthma.

Tejas is Fire. Prana inflames Tejas in the same way that a bellows inflames a hearth fire. When the mind is stable and discrimination is strong Tejas burns cleanly and purely and is transferred efficiently to the body. When motion or inertia affects the mind, or discrimination is agitated by memory or swamped by emotion, Tejas is perverted. Then its transfer into the body produces greater amounts of Pitta. Since consciousness is strongly influenced by chemical toxins transported by blood, the ability of Tejas to properly nourish the physical digestion depends on blood, on the liver and spleen, which control blood, and on the brain.

Ojas is the medium through which the force of Tejas is transmitted. Both physical and mental digestion can be strong only when Ojas is strong. Ojas and Kapha are closely related. When there is good digestion of food and other sensory impressions Ojas is efficiently produced. Weakened digestion causes increased Kapha production, and promotes production of ama.

Ojas is a substance, unlike Tejas and Prana, which means that it can be produced, collected and stored. Anything which increases Vata decreases Ojas, including dry or stale food, excessive exposure to wind and sun, worry, fear, sorrow, old age, fasting from sleep, and excessive loss of any body tissue. Loss of Shukra, which nourishes Ojas directly, is more detrimental than loss of other tissues. This is one reason why sexual restraint is recommended in Ayurveda.

Ama is the sinister counterpart of Ojas. Ojas is a living force that protects the integrity of the individual. Ama is a living force in the sense that it is a rich broth of nutrients for any alien invaders like bacteria, viruses and cancer cells who might choose to try to subjugate the system.

When Ojas is strong Tejas can properly digest and assimilate food and nourish all the dhatus, which strengthens ahamkara and your identity. A strong central identity will not allow either ama or intruders to remain in the system. Weak Ojas interferes with the transmission of Tejas, which weakens the digestion and encourages production of ama. Ama is useful nutrition only for intruders, and weakens both the dhatus and ahamkara. A weak ahamkara in turn encourages alien identities to flourish in the muck of ama, just as a weak government encourages the proliferation of lawlessness.

Ojas is the foundation of your physical immunity, and produces your aura. Your aura is your first line of defense against intrusions from the outside, a buffer against all the negativity that is consciously and unconsciously projected against you each day. Weak Ojas allows more negativity to seep through the aura barrier, increasing internal disharmony. The weaker your aura, the less stress you can simply shrug off and ignore.

Indigestion

Indigestion is the base of all physical diseases, the condition from which all other disease conditions arise. In a sense indigestion, the inability of an individual to digest any physical, mental or emotional input, is the sole disease of living beings. It usually begins in the mind as a "offense against wisdom," and is projected from the mind into the physical body.

All disease results from a combination of physical, mental and spiritual causes. Some diseases like ulcerative colitis are mainly due to mental influences; others like the common cold are mainly physical. Patients who suffer from both a mental and a physical disease, such as schizophrenia and asthma, or psychosis and arthritis, usually find that the physical problem gets worse whenever the mental disorder goes into remission and vice versa. Ultimately all diseases are mental; all are caused by willfulness, that perversion of intellect and common sense which makes us do what we are not supposed to do. This willful perversity is *prajnaparadha,* "offense against wisdom."

For example, suppose you are a VK person living in northern Minnesota. It is the middle of the night in the middle of winter and a blizzard is blowing outside. You are suddenly struck by a craving for ice cream. You know that ice cream is cold, wet, sticky, heavy and Kapha-producing, and that both night and winter are Kapha times, and that your constitution has Kapha in it. You know that if you eat the ice cream you are begging to increase Kapha, but you do it anyway, and the next morning your system is thoroughly clogged with Kapha. This is your "punishment" for a "offense against wisdom." It is not punishment in the classic sense; no one sits on high throwing thunderbolts at us for eating the wrong food. This sort of penalty occurs automatically when one of the rules of healthy living is violated. As an astute Indian woman once said, we are punished not *for* our actions but *by* our actions; each of our "offenses against wisdom" seeds the reaction that follows.

Transcontinental airplane flight is a stress to anyone regardless of constitution. You can travel across the United States in about six hours, crossing three time zones in the process. Your consciousness arrives at your destination in six hours and accompanies you off the plane. Your body, however, does not really arrive until three days later, since it takes about a day for it to recover from each time zone you cross. If you take the time to rest and recuperate from your journey you can adapt easily to your new location.

Your mind, however, hates to remain still, and does not like to permit the body to remain still. It often convinces itself that its balance is contingent on getting pending work out of the way as quickly as possible. Intercontinental air travel is a stress, and so is trying to go to work as soon as you land. Your mind's impatience with your body over its jetlag strain further impedes the adaptation process. If your mind gets its way and you try to go about business as usual there is a good chance that your body will sulk, and will express its displeasure by becoming ill. You cannot blame your body for taking revenge on your mind; your illness is a natural product of your "offense against wisdom."

The mind's physiology parallels that of the body. Like the physical Five Great Elements the mind has its own Five Elements:

Stability, the mental equivalent of Earth;

Emotion, the mental equivalent of Water;

Discrimination, the mental equivalent of Fire;

Memory, the mental equivalent of Air; and

Emptiness, the mental equivalent of Space.

Emptiness of mind is that which permits the other states of mind to manifest. Discrimination is the mind's digestion, which determines whether or not a course of action is appropriate for the well being of the organism. As long as your power of discrimination functions normally you will turn away from committing "offenses against wisdom." Mental instability weakens your ability to discriminate, just as disturbance of Vata, Pitta and Kapha affect the physical body's digestive capacity. Weak discrimination encourages the formation of mental ama (abnormal perceptions), just as weak digestion allows physical ama (toxic wastes) to be produced.

Vata, Pitta and Kapha are in charge of uniting the Five Great Physical Elements together in the body. Sattva, Rajas and Tamas perform the same function for the mind. Healthful, simple, well-digested food and healthful, simple habits promote Sattva. Intense, stimulating foods and intense activities like sex promote Rajas. Stale, putrid food and dulling activities like sleep promote Tamas. Rajas and Tamas are the doshas of the mind. They are needed in small quantities, but cause disease when they accumulate to excess.

Good physical digestion is associated with these signs:

1. You feel no discomfort after ingesting your desired quantity of food.

2. After eating you do not burp gas which has the same odor and taste as the food you ate.

3. Your stomach does not feel full for an unusual length of time after your meal.

4. No symptoms are produced as the food passes through your small intestine and colon; you should not even be aware of this stage of digestion.

5. You excrete your feces at your habitual time. It must be of the proper consistency and should have no blood, mucus or undigested food in it, nor should it be offensive in odor.

6. After digestion your physical desire for food returns at the usual hour. (A mental desire for gratification of the tongue does not count.)

If any of the above is lacking, physical indigestion is present.

Good mental digestion is associated with these signs:

1. You feel no mental discomfort after ingesting your desired quantity of sense objects.

2. Your mind does not feel full and jaded afterwards, nor does it "burp up" any reactions to what you experienced.

3. No untoward emotions are produced while you are processing this new information.

4. You are able to effortlessly and accurately retrieve your experience from memory and communicate it on demand.

5. Your sleep after indulgence is sound and enjoyable, and free of disturbing dreams (which are indicative of mental ama).

6. Desire for further sensory gratification arises after an appropriate period of time.

If any of the above is lacking, mental indigestion is present.

Physical indigestion can cause mental indigestion, and vice versa, but most often the two exist together. Since the body is much easier to control than the mind Ayurveda teaches that it is best to purify and balance the body first, to whatever extent possible, before turning to address the mind. A harmonized body exerts a harmonizing effect on the mind.

Physical indigestion is basically of three types: that caused by Vata, that caused by Pitta, and that caused by Kapha. Any one of these doshas can cause the body to lose its ability to process food, each in a different way. We can know by the symptoms produced which dosha is predominantly disturbed.

Vata-caused indigestion mainly affects the large intestine. Constipation alternates with loose stools, and there is usually copious intestinal gas, but all symptoms are variable. For a few days digestion improves, and then for no apparent reason the old symptoms return. The situation is so ever-changing that the individual does not know what to eat or when to eat to produce the unpredictable intermittent spells of good digestion.

Pitta-caused indigestion affects mainly the small intestine, and usually causes loose stools. Sensations of heat heartburn or anal burning after defecation are common. The patient may crave hot spicy food, which if consumed only worsens the condition.

Kapha-caused indigestion affects mainly the stomach. The sufferer usually feels no desire for food at all, and may complain of heaviness in the upper abdomen, watering of the mouth, and heaviness in the limbs. Constipation is common.

Kapha is most at home in the stomach, Pitta in the small intestine, and Vata in the colon. If indigestion is allowed to continue untreated one or more of these doshas will increase greatly, leave its home organ, and begin to circulate in the system searching for a weak area in which it can locate and cause a disease. Untreated indigestion thus results in acute diseases like colds, fevers, coughs, influenza, diarrhea, peptic ulcer, and so on. All these diseases are methods Nature uses to purify your organism when your being has failed to "digest" its life experiences well and has instead allowed physical and mental filth to collect inside you.

No matter how efficiently you treat an acute disease your effort will be wasted unless you also address the underlying indigestion. Until you eliminate this root other diseases will sprout from it. When possible treatment should begin with the uprooting of the root cause of the disease, after which any specific manifestations can be rectified. Life-threatening situations require emergency attention, true, but once the crisis passes the indigestion remains to be tackled

Ayurvedic Treatment

A Yogi named Chaitanyananda lived about 200 miles from Bombay until his death not long ago. His cures of serious diseases, extending even to the first stages of cancer, were well documented, and people flocked from all over India to receive treatment at his hands.

He would welcome with profuse greetings anyone who came to him, to create in them a false sense of security. While they rested he would go into the jungle to collect a certain herb whose juice was then administered to the unsuspecting patient. About fifteen minutes later the poor sufferer would begin to vomit and purge. This vigorous purification would last for up to three hours. After the nausea and diarrhea died down the exhausted patient would receive a bowl of split mung beans and rice cooked together into the preparation known as *khichadi*. Into this porridge Chaitanyananda would add a mixture of *bhasmas* (mineral and metallic oxides) in a specific proportion according to the nature of the disease. After repeating this process for thirty days the patient was clean from top to bottom, and the disease had usually disappeared.

Chaitanyananda never studied classical Ayurveda in a college, but his treatment followed Ayurvedic lines:

Remove the cause.
Purify, to eliminate excess doshas.
Balance the doshas and rekindle the digestive fire.
Rejuvenate, to rebuild the organism.

No therapy that fails to balance the doshas is Ayurvedic, or likely to be permanently effective. Even when the mind is unbalanced that imbalance is either due to dosha imbalance or is made worse by it.

The single most powerful dosha-rebalancing, fire-enkindling, rejuvenating force in the universe is faith. Recall that one symptom of diseased Rasa Dhatu is "lack of faith." Faith in Nature and Her ability to cure actively strengthens Rasa Dhatu, which then nourishes the other dhatus, and Ojas. Faith enhances ahamkara's ability to self-identify with the body, and strengthens the bond between the individual and his or her cosmos. Faith in healing is the key to health.

Vimalananda always said that there are only two ways to cure a disease. You can have faith in another being—a physician, a deity, your grandmother, or anyone else—and put yourself entirely in his or her hands, allowing that person to direct the force of your faith. Otherwise you must have faith in yourself, in your own powers of self-healing, and heal yourself directly.

Faith was an important ingredient in Chaitanyananda's cures. People came to him expecting relief because they had heard tales of all those whom he had helped, and this faith helped cure them. If you have no Chaitanyananda to force you to become healthy you become responsible for curing yourself. Then you will have to decide, with all parts of your being, that you are so tired of being unbalanced that you are prepared to undergo patiently whatever discipline may be necessary to heal yourself. Until you can say to yourself sincerely that you are ready to change your ways your healing cannot occur. A firm decision to heal yourself only happens when your mind is ready to admit to willfulness and "offenses against wisdom," when it is willing to admit to its deviousness in blaming the body for its own excesses. When your mind is truly contrite, and willing to forgive itself for falling ill, it is sure to cooperate with your body to do the job right.

Hopelessness or helplessness is dangerous because it deprives your immune system of support from ahamkara. If your mind decides that it is fed up with any body part, that body part is likely to lose its immunity and become quickly devitalized. Be angry, be hostile, experience any emotion that wants to come out, but never fall prey to hopelessness if you want to be cured.

Moreover, you have to want everyone to be healthy if you want to become healthy. Nature's Law mandates that you get back whatever you put out. You will receive health only if your activities and attitudes promote, or at least do not interfere with, the health of those around you. Like disease, health is contagious; it can be passed from one person to another, again and again.

Above all, be patient. Why do you think people who are ill are called "patients"? Patience is not resignation, an emotion that is usually best reserved for your deathbed. Too often resignation implies paralysis or surrender on ahamkara's part just at the moment when ahamkara's energy most needs to be mobilized. Patience is a virtue because it represents ahamkara's admission of willingness to do whatever must be done over whatever period of time to achieve your goal of renewed well-being.

The discussions below outline some aspects of the Ayurvedic management of certain conditions. They do not purport to be a guide to self-treatment of serious diseases. Self-help is the best help only when you are sure of what you are doing. Until then always seek expert professional guidance for any serious disorder.

Elimination of Ama

When your tongue is coated, your feces foul, and your urine turbid ama is present in your digestive tract, It must first be removed before anything else is done. The best way to do this is to do nothing: allow the body to expel the ama on its own, by fasting.

Fasting is called in Ayurveda the first and best of all medicines. When possible you should fast for 24 to 48 hours on as little of anything as possible. If you are acutely ill, as with a fever, this should not be too difficult; you probably will not want anything anyway. Brew up some weak tea of dried ginger (_ to 1 tsp. per quart of water, boil for 20 minutes) and sip it, just enough to prevent dehydration. Add a few drops of lemon juice if you like. As soon as your urine, feces and tongue clear, your digestive tract is free of acute ama and purification can proceed. If you are not acutely ill, 24 to 48 hours on weak ginger tea may seem like an eternity if you are a V or a P. In such cases you can provide your body some additional substance, in the form of thin rice gruel, while it works to empty itself of ama.

Once the ama has exited your digestive tract you must ensure that Vata, Pitta and Kapha flow freely again. This is the province of the therapies known collectively as *panchakarma,* the "Five Actions": emesis, purgation, enema, nasal medication, and bloodletting. Emesis, or therapeutic vomiting, is the best way to improve flow when Kapha congestion has been the main cause of your disease. Purgation eliminates Pitta accumulation, and enema controls Vata. Nasal medication works on doshas accumulated in the head, and bloodletting purifies Blood directly.

Ayurveda regards medicated enema as the most important purification method of all, because of the importance of the large intestine in health and disease. Judiciously medicated enemas work both to control ama and to facilitate the absorption of Prana.

Your system must be well prepared before you undergo panchakarma. Specifically you must:

1. *Determine which of your doshas is most disturbed.* Usually your state of indigestion can tell you. Also consider your constitution, and this axiom:

There is no *pain* without involvement of Vata.

There is no *inflammation* without involvement of Pitta.

There is no *pus formation* without involvement of Kapha.

Whenever there is intense pain, especially colicky or stabbing in nature, Vata is present. Whenever fever or inflammation predominate, as in an ulcer, Pitta is in excess. Whenever there is pus formation anywhere, even in the sputum as in bronchitis, Kapha is disturbed.

2. *Oil your body.* When your body is relatively purified you can use any oil that agrees with your constitution and condition. Whenever your body is full of ama, however, ordinary oils will create additional congestion. In such cases you should only use castor oil, applying it externally to any areas that are painful or inflamed due to ama. You can also use it internally, in the dose of 1 Tbsp. with a cup of strong tea made of powdered ginger, to scrape ama away from the tissues.

3. *Sweat.* Sweat is oil's partner in Vata control. Thermography shows that painful areas in the body where there is no inflammation are often several degrees cooler than normal. This sort of pain is the result of constricted blood vessels. One of the effects which painkilling drugs show is a temporary restoration to normal temperatures of these painful parts. Such cold may have a physical cause, or it may be due to fear and other cold emotions, or both. To warm yourself up use dry heat, like saunas or burying yourself under heavy blankets, exclusively whenever there is any body obstruction due to ama. When there is little ama you can use wet heat, like steam baths or hot tubs. Normally you should not apply direct heat to your eyes, heart or testicles.

4. *Purify.* Oil and heat "soften up" your system, helping to mobi-

lize all the ancient ama trapped in your dhatus so that it can be excreted. Ayurveda's texts use this analogy: A dried stick is so brittle that it breaks when it is bent, whereas if you first soak the stick in oil and then warm it gently it will regain its suppleness, and again be able to bend without breaking. You must similarly be careful to avoid "bending" your body with panchakarma before adequately heating and oiling it, lest it be damaged.

All purification measures must be used with care, for they can cause side-effects when improperly administered. Purification must not be done during any extremes of climate—heat waves, cold snaps, flash floods, wind storms—and is forbidden to the very young, the very old, the very weak, and pregnant women.

In general:

When the patient is strong and the disease is weak, use panchakarma directly

When the patient is weak and the disease is strong, strengthen the patient and weaken the disease before doing panchakarma.

Panchakarma is not heroics. Like all other Ayurvedic therapies it emulates Nature's methods to assist Her in healing the individual. Here is an example: some years ago I was helping a friend of mine perform some emergency maintenance on the brakes of his car. We were in Northern Ontario. It was early spring. Assuming that the work would be done quickly we postponed lunch.

We ended up spending almost five hours on the repairs. In the late afternoon, the Vata time of day, a chill wind blew up, which did nothing to improve our exasperation over the delay in the process. Eventually we got home, disappointed that we had missed our chance to go canoeing. Within half an hour of our arrival, my friend was down with a fever.

I knew it was due to Vata. It had arisen quickly, a characteristic of many Vata diseases. The causative factors were all Vata-producing: strenuous exertion leading to fatigue, cold wind, hunger, exasperation, late afternoon, and disappointment creating Bitterness. I told him to eat some fresh khichadi with ghee, to replenish the nutrients he had burned off by his exertion, and then to accompany me to the sauna, to allow its heat to control Vata's cold. While heat is not good for Pitta-type fevers it is sometimes appropriate for those due to Vata or Kapha.

He did as I suggested, and after a few moments in the heat became nauseated and had to leave to go vomit. I regarded this as a good sign: the khichadi had attracted the Vata to the stomach, the ghee had oiled his insides, and the sweat had facilitated Vata's movement. He returned to the sauna feeling much relieved, collected more heat, vomited once again, and went to bed. The next morning, after a good rest, he was as good as new. This procedure, which only helped Nature do what She wanted to do, would not work in every case, of course, but was just right for his.

TRIPHALA

Panchakarma is a wonderful thing, but it is only a beginning. If you have been mistreating your body for many years you have many layers of ama to be removed. Each layer must be loosened before it can be expelled. Even if you could eliminate all ama at once it would be unwise to do so; if your organs of elimination were unable to process all those toxins your system could become seriously disordered.

Besides, your organism has had these toxins in it so long that it has developed a metabolic equilibrium that involves them. Feeling its metabolic rug being pulled from underneath it, it will resist all revolutionary changes, particularly if a mass of fear-producing Vata has accumulated within you. Chaitanyananda avoided this problem by providing an environment of complete stability and security that his guests could use as a haven while their worlds were being turned inside out. If you can retire to such a refuge for at least six weeks when you purify, fine; otherwise you will be wise to follow each spell of purification with weeks of balancing the doshas and nourishing the dhatus.

Panchakarma is a depletive procedure (called *apatarpana* in Sanskrit), and all depletion tends to weaken ahamkara. Inadequate *santarpana* (rebuilding the dhatus) after panchakarma is bound to weaken your immunity. Colonics may be beneficial for ridding the body of impurities, for example, but if they are overused they will cause severe Vata disturbance as they deplete the system without offering anything in return. Aggravated Vata will produce such cellular fear that the system will then actually hold onto any remaining ama with increased tenacity. Your system must be confidently willing to release its stored toxins if your purifications are to be successful. Slow and steady in purification is always best.

Excess in purification can actually drive ama deeper into your tissues. Overuse of Hot, Pungent foods or herbs like garlic and cayenne, excessive exercise, and repression of emotions are as likely to disturb the purification process as are more obvious violations of purification like restraint of natural urges, improper food combining, and indulgence in stimulants like alcohol or caffeine. You must be careful to purify at your system's preferred rate of speed, no matter how boring that pace may seem to your impatient mind.

As Triphala gradually, gently purifies and rejuvenates your digestive tract, it improves your ability to nourish your dhatus. Triphala, which literally means "three fruits," is composed of three unique herbs: amalaki, haritaki and bibhitaki. Though amalaki's main Taste is Sour its secondary Tastes are Sweet, Bitter, Pungent and Astringent. Its Energy is Cold, and its Post-Digestive Effect is Sweet. It balances all Three Doshas but is best for controlling Pitta. Amalaki's Sour Taste can improve the digestive fire without disturbing Pitta thanks to its Sweet Post-Digestive Effect and Cold Energy. Fresh amalaki fruit is intensely Sour, but when you drink a glass of water after eating an amalaki the water tastes as sweet as syrup.

One amalaki the size of a plum contains many times the vitamin C of an orange. This vitamin C apparently exists in a heat-stable form that enables most of it to survive the cooking or drying processes used during the fruit's preparation. Amalaki is a superior rejuvenator; one of its Sanskrit names is "Wet-Nurse," in honor of the care with which it, like sleep, improves body and mind. It is used therapeutically in a wide range of conditions, but particularly for hyperacidity and liver complaints. It is also used in shampoos, and oil medicated with it improves the hair and brain.

Haritaki's main Taste is Astringent, but it is secondarily Sweet, Sour, Bitter and Pungent. It has Hot Energy and Sweet Post-Digestive Effect. It balances all Three Doshas but is best for Vata because it can consolidate the body and mind with its Astringency while controlling Vata via Sweet and Hot. It scrapes old adherent ama from the digestive tract and tones the colon.

Bibhitaki's main Taste is also Astringent, with secondary Sweet, Bitter and Pungent. Its Energy is Hot and its Post-digestive Effect Sweet. It balances all Three Doshas but is best for Kapha, being predominantly Astringent and Hot. It purifies all body fluids and is especially useful in asthma.

Triphala is the Ayurvedic panacea. You can use it to wash your hair or body, or as a laxative, purgative, or emetic, or in an enema. Its decoction can be used as eye, nose or ear drops, or for gargling. It scrapes toxins from body tissues and causes doshas that have left their proper locations—stomach, small intestine, and colon—to return there. Because of its powerful ability to purify it is also used to detoxify substances like metals before they are prepared into medicines. Triphala is harmless, but very toxic persons sometimes react if they use too large a dose too soon in their detoxification. Triphala can mobilize stored toxins faster than a weakened system can process them, which can sometimes lead to a skin rash as the body tries to throw the excess of the toxins out through the skin. If such a rash develops when you begin using Triphala stop it immediately, let the rash disappear and then begin it again, taking half the dose you had taken previously.

The best way to use Triphala powder for gradual purification and regeneration of the digestive tract is to stir 1 tsp. of it into a glass of pure water and let it sit overnight. Next morning drink the water without stirring, allowing the sediment to remain on the bottom, then refill the glass and stir vigorously. Let it sit all day long, and drink it again at night without stirring. Then discard the dregs and stir a fresh teaspoonful into a fresh glass of water for the next day.

If this is too laxative a dose or if it causes some reaction drink only one glass daily. Let the refilled glass stand all day and all night, drink it the next morning, and after discarding the remains prepare a fresh mixture for the next morning. In this way 1 tsp. will last you for two days. If this still causes a reaction, reduce the amount to 1/2 tsp. Once you find your proper dose continue this routine for three to six months for maximum benefit. You can repeat it regularly if need be.

FASTING

Ayurveda frowns on long-term fasting. The sense of deprivation that a long fast creates can encourage ahamkara to demand a long spell of indulgence afterward, to rebuild her confidence. I once knew a Westerner in India who had decided to fast his way to enlightenment. He being an extreme example of the V constitution I knew how dangerous this would be and warned him pointedly about the possible perils. It was impossible to change his mind, though; he obstinately ignored all warnings. One day his starving, devitalized immune system landed him in the hospital, where doctors lanced a long abscess running all the way up his leg. The outcome of this adventure into higher consciousness? After his recovery he returned to North America and became a cook!

His persistent fasting so starved his dhatus that they eventually overwhelmed his resolve. This cycle of overrestriction followed by overgratification aggravates Vata in nearly everyone who attempts it. To fast regularly for one day every week or two is far better for the body than to fast and then to binge. Your digestive organs need a regular day off as much as you do, and it does them little good to make them work overtime without any rest for months at a stretch and then give them a long enforced fasting vacation.

During an illness you should fast as long as you have no real desire for food. As long as you feel lighter, brighter and healthier without food, continue your fast. As soon as you begin to lose your energy and feel real hunger, consume well-cooked rice or barley gruel until that also fails to satisfy your appetite. Then switch to khichadi, the preparation of rice and split mung beans the recipe for which is given in the Appendix. Khichadi, which purifies and nourishes the dhatus, is an ideal diet during prolonged therapy of any chronic disease. It eliminates both mental and physical ama as it relaxes and lightens the mind.

Fasting should be used as a purification only if panchakarma cannot be done, which means that daily enemas and other such heroic procedures should form no part of your fast. If you do choose to fast for a prolonged period and have never fasted before you should get professional guidance beforehand. You may experience acute physical stress if your system begins to mobilize ama faster than your organs of excretion can handle it.

You should also follow the restrictions applicable to your constitution. V people, for example, should not fast on water or any other severely restricted diet for more than a day or two. Absolute fasting for as little as a week can wreck metabolic balance in a V that may have taken months to obtain. V types should select instead a single food, like khichadi, on which they can live for a month or more at a time.

P people can fast on liquids like fruit or vegetable juices or on raw fruits and vegetables, but not on water alone. They should not skimp on quantity. K people alone may indulge in a prolonged water fast if they so desire. Otherwise, they may use raw juices. K people in particular need to develop a regular weekly fasting habit, to promote strong digestion.

V people may fast once weekly or bi-monthly on liquids other than water alone. Some Vs like lemon juice and honey in pure water; others enjoy juices, and those who are not allergic to dairy may prefer milk, fresh whey, or yogurt blended with water. None of these should be refrigerator cold. Ps can use diluted fruit juices, like grape, prune or pomegranate, or Bitter or Astringent vegetable juices like cucumber. They should avoid Sour juices. K types should avoid juices that are either intensely Sweet or Sour.

Balancing the Doshas

Whether or not you have used panchakarma for purification you must focus your healing process on balancing your unbalanced doshas.

If you have a V constitution, or if your indigestion and ama formation were due to Vata, you may use:

Dry ginger, fennel, or dill to digest ama.

Lemon, lime or grapefruit for the Sour Taste, rock salt for the Salty Taste, and ginger or garlic for the Pungent Taste to rekindle your digestion. Medicinal wines are excellent for the V digestive fire.

Light, well-cooked food and warm liquids, especially with ginger added.

Mild exercise, especially simple Yoga stretches; regular sunbathing; and indirect ventilation, since strong winds increase Vata.

If Pitta caused your problem, you may use:

Fennel to digest ama. You may use dry ginger if it is not too intense for you.

Psyllium seed husks, Triphala, or any Bitter herb like gentian to rekindle your digestion.

Light or raw foods and juices with cold coriander or sandalwood tea.

Strolling in the open air, especially near flowing water; moderate sunbathing, early or late in the day; and regular exposure to wind to help dry Pitta.

If Kapha caused your problem, you may use:

Dry ginger, black pepper or cumin to digest ama.

Any Bitter or Pungent herbs like garlic or black pepper to enkindle the digestive fire.

Small quantities of food, especially roasted, with as little liquid as possible; tea of dry ginger is best.

Vigorous exercise; extensive sunbathing, well-wrapped if need be to encourage sweating; and windbathing, well wrapped to preserve body heat.

Psyllium seed husks, known as isabgol or flea-seed husks in India, are an excellent way to purify the intestines. If they are being used to absorb excess water from the body they should be taken dry, otherwise they should first be soaked in some liquid to prevent them from causing constipation and congestion. If you are not allergic to dairy you can soak psyllium husks in milk to relieve constipation or in a blend of yogurt and water to relieve loose stools.

Regular use of psyllium, which is heavy for digestion, can over a long period weaken the V or K digestive fire. You can prevent this by consuming an ounce of a medicinal wine diluted with an ounce of water at the same time that you take the psyllium. Until Ayurvedic medicinal wines become readily available you can use instead an ounce of organic additive-free wine diluted with an ounce of water, or half a cup of tea made of dry ginger.

Even after you quit using medicines your dietary control must continue for at least six weeks, as must your restrictions on your normal habits of indulgence. Ayurveda's texts list eight common practices which can recreate a disease in those who are healing:

- Excessive and forceful talking
- Travelling, especially long distance
- Excessive walking
- Continual sitting or lying in one position
- Overeating leading to indigestion
- Inappropriate diet with improper food combining
- Sleeping during the day (except in summer); and
- Any kind of sexual activity.

Mental Medication

Balancing Vata is sure to reduce fear but cannot eliminate it entirely, especially in an individual with a V constitution, whose very genes possess the potential to create fear. Fear is always intensified and worsened by worry, and a recuperating V person should be kept occupied and never be given time to worry. Meditation is the best occupation, the only direct way to eliminate fear. Exercise or a hobby may be useful if it sufficiently intriguing to induce the individual to concentrate on it. Vs must however guard against the addiction that they can develop to any kind of active recreation. Passive pursuits like listening to music, or even enjoying spectator sports, are also addictive but their passive nature is less likely to exhaust a V.

Likewise, anger can only be reduced, not eliminated, in a P individual, who has anger-creating genes. Impatience, which produces anger or jealousy, is the key disturbance in the P individual. Since impatience usually occurs when the mind is idle, the P mind should always have something to work on. Mere pastimes will not suffice, as they may for Vata, because Pitta needs problems to gnaw on, things to "digest" and solve little by little. Difficult problems are good, since Ps will usually stay with a project until it is finished, but not a moment longer. Most any sort of complicated project that is beneficial to the individual will do.

K people have complacency in their genes. Treatment of Kapha-caused indigestion can only control it, not eliminate it. Complacency may manifest as greed to consume and possess whatever one can obtain, or it may indicate a lackadaisical attitude toward health. The Earth in Kapha tends to set K people stubbornly in their ways. Vigorous motivation, by self or others, is the only way to balance these traits. It is best to concentrate on one activity in the beginning. Though it may take quite a while, once a K individual becomes dedicated to self-improvement his or her inertial force will cause the progression to continue, though without periodic "booster" doses of motivation it may gradually slow to a halt again.

Our ability to act on our intentions is limited by our capacity to integrate them into ourselves. A sattvic person, who has an abundance of mental equilibrium or Sattva, comprehends well and follows his or her path steadily and consistently, and progresses quickly. Full as they are of the hyperactivity of Rajas, Rajasic people twist facts to fit their preconceptions, and convince themselves that they are progressing when they are in fact merely reinforcing ahamkara's dependencies. Tamasic people, whose abundant inert Tamas guides their being, ignore clear evidence of the need to progress and dig in where they are in hope of remaining there.

Mental digestion predominates over physical digestion. If you bite off more than you can chew, be it a book you are writing or a cake you are eating, you do so because of weakness of ahamkara. When she is weak but believes herself to be strong she may try to prove it with overambition. If your mind is relatively clear this self-delusion will be temporary and you will remove the "food" from your "mouth" before you try to chew it up.

If you tenaciously hold onto your "food" and try determinedly to chew it up you will be chewing up more than you can swallow. You can still spit out the "food" whenever you admit to your self-deception, but the longer you hold onto it the more ahamkara invests in displaying to the world that she can do whatever she sets out to do. Allowing ahamkara's investment in her assumed persona to regulate your life causes you to swallow more than you can digest.

At this stage you can prevent undigested experience from entering your system by "vomiting" it: making a clean breast of the affair and admitting to a "offense against wisdom." If you fail to do this physical or mental ama will be created and absorbed into your system, at which point some disease or another becomes inevitable.

A friend of mine once opened a school for herbal studies, and permitted his ambition to overwhelm his mental digestion. He enrolled fifteen students, both because he needed their fees to break even and because he felt he was strong enough to teach them all adequately. As the term progressed he found himself overwhelmed by the needs of these fifteen diverse individuals, and began to overwork. His ability to follow through could not keep pace with his intentions. In his enthusiasm to empower others by transferring his knowledge to them he was ruining his own health.

The stress of continuously having to adapt to fifteen different ahamkaras depressed his digestion and created mental ama. Because he would not at first admit to himself that he had overextended his limits he buried that ama inside himself. For self-protection his mind projected the imbalance into his body. When last we met he was complaining of symptoms which suggested a disturbed gall bladder.

His diet was appropriate for his constitution, and the season was not Pitta aggravating, so clearly his problems were mainly based in his mind. As we conversed he himself made the connection between imperfect mental digestion and weakness of a physical digestive organ, and realized that he needed to eliminate the indigestible situation which was causing his problem. He could do this either by decreasing his student load or by enlisting assistance to help him with it. His recognition of the problem ensured that he would be able to solve it.

Management of mental disorders involves essentially the same steps outlined for physical treatment. When poor mental digestion has created many untoward emotions and the accumulation of those emotions eventually distorts the self-image and the ability to function efficiently, removal of the cause is the first requisite. Next, the mind must be purified. Mental inertia requires strenuous stimulation to induce it to purify. A mind filled with anger releases that anger readily, purifying itself somewhat thereby. But a mind filled with fear holds tenaciously to its fear, and releases it only after mental heat and oil, which is sincere affection (Sneha), have been applied to it consistently.

Of course, when an individual's mind is weak and the disorder is strong purification is usually unwise, as it will further weaken the mind. While shock therapy (under competent professional supervision only!) is indicated in selected cases, slow and deliberate balancing of Rajas and Tamas with the help of the power of Sattva is usually the therapy of choice. Mental rejuvenation is indicated in all cases.

Fasting from cravings is a must when the mind has become filled with ama created from unsatisfactory interpersonal relationships. There is even a mental Triphala to help scrape away the old ama of selfish attachments. It is called *kirtana*, the devotional singing of God's name. Even if you don't believe in a God with form you can select a name which represents whatever you do believe in and repeat it with devotion, allowing that force to enter and heal you.

Kirtana, which helps us rectify our relationship with Nature, is the best of all rejuvenators. The true meaning of Yoga is union with the divine, and an attitude of sincere request for divine assistance is the royal road to real Yoga.

Yukti

The word *yukti* is derived from the same root as the word Yoga. Yukti is defined in Sanskrit as *bahu-karana-yoga-ja*: created from the union of many causes. The traditional example for the action of yukti is the production of a clay pot. A pot is a union of clay, water, a wheel, a stick to form the pot, a kiln to fire it, fuel for the kiln, and a potter to oversee the entire process.

Yukti also produces health. One person's cancer may disappear after treatment with powerful medicines, another's may recede after visualizations alone, and a third's may respond exclusively to diet. Cure depends on a therapy that may be more or less complex, a patient who must have faith in something, individuals who will administer the therapies to the patient, and a director to oversee. Above all the director must be competent. Someone, be it the patient, a relative, a friend or a professional, needs to know what to do and when to do it. It is said that even if the remedy is insufficient, the assistants are incompetent and the patient is recalcitrant a skillful therapist can still provide relief, using the principle of yukti to combine removal of the cause, purification, balancing and rejuvenation into one harmonious whole therapy.

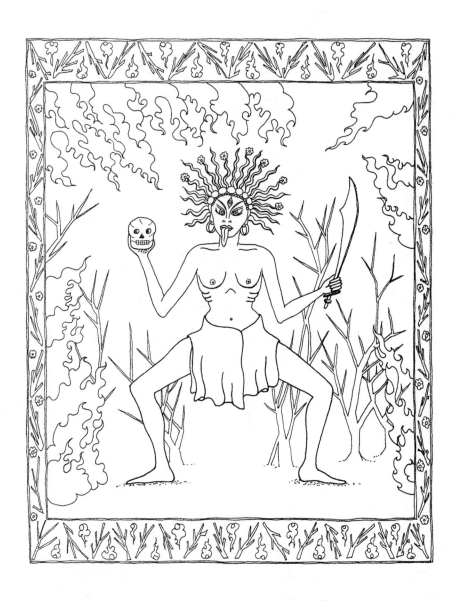

Chapter Seven
Disease

Without yukti, the adept combining of attitude and activity for individual harmonization, indigestion tends to become chronic and mutate into new forms. Chronic indigestion weakens and sensitizes the immune system, which reacts first with allergy, then auto-immune disease. Finally conditions like cancer or AIDS supervene in which immunity collapses altogether. Weakness of ahamkara's self-identification with the body is the root cause of all such conditions.

Allergy

An antigen is anything, usually but not always a protein, which can be recognized as being foreign to the organism. Ama is a general term for any substance that is unwilling or unable to cooperate with ahamkara's plans for you. Every piece of improperly digested food that gets absorbed into your system becomes ama. Much of the ama in your body acts as antigenic ("antibody-stimulating") material and induces your immune system to produce antibodies to it. Each antibody binds tightly to its chosen antigen, and if your immune system is healthy it completes this policing job by sweeping the antibody-antigen complexes from your being.

Antibodies are specialized proteins that your body makes to order when exposed to a particular antigen. The more antigens you are exposed to, the greater the variety of antibodies you will produce. It has been estimated that by adulthood most of us have antibodies to more than 100 million foreign (ama) molecules. Usually your immune system classifies this ama according to its source: cheese ama, pork ama, peanut ama, and so on.

When you are exposed over and over again to the same ama you will produce more and more antibodies to it as your system steels itself against each wave of invasion. If you know that you do not digest peanuts well and yet you persistently, perversely consume them, those imperfectly digested peanuts will persistently form ama. Eventually so much peanut ama will accumulate in you that whenever a peanut touches your lips or tongue your immune police will sound an alarm, assuming that this peanut too will be improperly digested. You discover that you have an allergy once this immune reaction becomes so pronounced that you are made aware of it, by some bodily or mental symptom produced as a side-effect of the internal combat.

Humans can become allergic to almost anything. Some people are allergic to mold, others to hydrocarbons and petrochemicals, still others to cat or dog hair, or mite feces. Some people break out into hives when they are exposed to sudden cold. There is even a condition called exercise-induced anaphylaxis in which strenuous exertion produces an allergic reaction that can be life-threatening. This, like the allergy to cold, is probably due to the toxic state of the organism rather than to a specific allergy to aerobics or frigidity. The sudden stress of cold or activity causes toxins to be mobilized from their tissue storage sites and flood the circulation.

An allergic reaction can cause almost any symptom. Acute disease with fever and/or pus is not likely to be allergic, nor are unilateral conditions (pains, swellings, and the like on one side of the body only). But the tendency to bilateral pains and swellings and to recurrent, repeated infections which might have pus and fever, like "chronic colds" and infections of the tonsils and ears, is often allergic.

Allergies occur in hypersensitive organisms. While specific allergies may respond to specific desensitization techniques, management of the overall allergic state requires that this generalized hypersensitivity be reduced. Vata and Pitta are the principal doshas involved in allergy, for it is their mutual intensity that oversensitizes the organism.

Allergies and sensitivity reactions are of many different varieties. Some occur only when you take the allergen often enough, for otherwise antibody levels do not build up high enough to induce a noticeable reaction. Others occur every time you consume a substance. The most insidious are the addictive allergies. As long as you take the substance you are allergic to, you feel fine; but as soon as you quit, you start to feel withdrawal symptoms.

Examining your cravings carefully can test this. Suppose you like to eat chocolate. If you crave it only occasionally and feel satisfied after a small piece you can be fairly confident that your body probably created that craving in you for some specific purpose. Perhaps it needed to balance itself out on that day with the help of some factor that is found in chocolate. It is a different matter if you feel out of sorts when you neglect to have your chocolate one day, or if you eat a small piece of chocolate and then suddenly experience an almost uncontrollable craving to consume all the chocolates in the box. These reactions suggest you have developed an addictive allergy to the chocolate. All addictions, even to the most virulent drugs, probably become allergic in nature with time.

The allergic tendency develops early in life, and is strongly influenced by prakriti. V and P types are much more commonly affected by allergy than are Ks. Some modern allergists note that most of their patients of food allergy are blond-haired and blue-eyed, people we can recognize as P, PV or PK types. One source has estimated that 30% of the American populace has some degree of food allergy.

In addition, after conception when the child is growing in the womb the mother sends some of her immune protection to her fetus across the placenta in the form of antibodies. If she is very toxic she may send too many antibodies along, or she may even transmit antigens circulating in her blood to her fetus. Immune reactions may thus begin in the baby's body even before birth.

For the first three months after birth the baby's delicate digestive tract absorbs lots of large molecules, including non-human proteins, which is one more reason why it is so important for newborns to get breast milk as long as possible. The mother's breast milk also provides passive immunity to the child—unless the mother eats an allergy-stimulating diet, in which case ama will enter her milk and the baby's immunity will suffer instead.

Allergies can also promote one another, and exposure to one substance may make you allergic to another. Allergy to alcohol, for example, which probably influences the development of both hangovers and alcoholism, may actually begin as allergy to the grain used in the fermentation process. Milk allergy may likewise develop from lactose intolerance, or it may begin as allergy to the antibiotics which are given to the cows as a disease preventative and then progress to allergy to the milk itself. Pork allergy may also begin as antibiotic sensitivity. Mass-produced chickens are fed many different drugs, all of which might sensitize the body against the chicken.

Intestinal toxemia is also involved in the development of allergy. Pollution in the large intestine permits irritating chemicals produced by improper digestion to inflame the membrane lining of the large intestine and reduce intestinal mobility. For example, improper digestion of the amino acid tyrosine produces the corrosive chemical phenol. One drop of pure phenol can burn a hole in your external skin; imagine its effect, even in diluted form, on the delicate internal "skin" (mucus membrane) that lines the digestive tract.

When this membrane is sufficiently damaged your gut begins to "leak," and your body begins to absorb substances which otherwise would be excreted. Toxins in food, metabolically produced toxins, and improperly digested fats, starches and proteins all act as ama. When absorbed into your system and carried via your circulation to other parts of your body these internal pollutants set up imbalances wherever they go.

"Leaky gut" is pervasive in our damaged society. Food allergies, modern medicines (including certain antibiotics and heavy doses of aspirin and ibuprofen), excessive drinking, parasitical infections, and compromised immune systems have all been implicated as causative factors. Modern researchers have found evidence of leaky gut in diabetics, alcoholics, smokers, burn patients, iron-deficient children, schizophrenics, and long-distance runners. Many other classes of people are likely to suffer from leaky gut to less-perceptible extents, accumulating ama more slowly and insidiously thereby. A few of the conditions that leaky gut can promote include insomnia, obesity, halitosis, asthma, arthritis, eczema, rashes, diarrhea, migraine and even depression.

Intestinal toxemia adversely affects brain and consciousness as well as body. Proper digestion of the amino acid tryptophan yields serotonin, the brain's "mellow chemical" which generally keeps us cool, calm and collected. Improper digestion of tryptophan produces indole and skatole, the chemicals that give feces its offensive odor. These agitate and disturb the brain. Tryptophan can temporarily calm the brain when it is ingested, but many of these temporarily calmed people will develop greater agitation over the long term from the chemicals they produce as a result of not digesting the tryptophan efficiently.

Abnormal processes also produce substances that are called "false neuro-transmitters," like octopamine. Such chemicals compete in the body with normal neurotransmitters, whose job is to accurately transfer messages across the brain. This competition leaves the consciousness even more scattered and disorganized, unable to properly monitor or maintain the organism's immune defenses.

Just as ama created from improper digestion of food can disturb the consciousness and agitate the emotions, disturbed emotions can themselves weaken the digestion and create physical ama, which can then incite an immune reaction. Deeply suppressed emotions can amplify allergic reactions, for as the mind feels threatened by its inability to express itself it tends to take out its frustrations on the substances that are invading it. A complete physical housecleaning would remedy the situation, though a deeply agitated mind will usually try to find solace in further for sensory indulgence rather than willingly submit to such purification. The continuous presence of ama in the system creates a condition of permanent immune alert, an allergic state.

Cantankerous Bowel Syndrome

The regular presence in the gut of indigestion and its resulting ama will sooner or later irritate it. If such irritation continues long enough the bowel will become chronically peevish, and will begin to resist cooperating with its organism even when its ambient conditions are generally agreeable.

Persistent bowel dysfunction occurs in many diseases, including diarrhea, dysentery, sprue, celiac disease, Crohn's disease, chronic colic, irritable bowel syndrome, "phantom" tumors (*gulma*), colitis, and ulcerative colitis. Ayurveda implicates it in the causation of hemorrhoids as well. All these conditions develop from weakness of the digestive fire, and their treatment requires re-enkindling the fires of mental and physical digestion alike. The restoratives discussed in the last chapter usually prove generally useful in such conditions, in particular Triphala, which is very nearly a panacea for imbalances of the digestion. But because these conditions have become chronic, have developed a physical and psychological momentum of their own, additional intervention is often required to return the organism to normal.

Perhaps the chief requirement for successfully treating a chronically irritated gut is patience, the taking of sufficient time to redress a condition that took time to develop. The overall causative dosha is of course Vata, which predominates in the ever-mobile, ever-changing digestive tract. All Vata-aggravating factors, from excessive exertion, fasting, sex, travel or late-night carousing to overuse of cold, dry, leftover, hard food, and destabilizing emotions like grief and fear, promote cantankerous bowel. Once Vata is aggravated it may act alone to create more problems, or may involve Pitta and Kapha in the pathology as well.

Treatment is according to predominant dosha. Vata aggravation is, for example, both the chief cause and the chief result of intestinal colic, a situation of spasm arisen in the bowel's muscles. Colic commonly responds readily to med-icinal wines, the application of herbal plasters (such as those of mustard seed and asafetida), the gentle binding of the abdomen, and/or the implant of oily enemata (1/2 cup of warm sesame oil, inserted gradually and retained for half an hour or more). Gulma, which is a painful swelling of the tissue of an abdom-inal organ with or without retention of its contents, is addressed similarly.

More commonly, though, Vata conspires with his fellow doshas to create sometimes-intricate patterns of digestive upset. Diarrhea and hemorrhoids tend to encourage one another to develop, and both can produce and/or develop from a condition of chronic "dysentery" which unlike the modern definition of dysentery need not be due to infection by some pathogen. Ayurveda calls "dysen-tery" any condition in which foul-smelling sticky, liquid or semi-solid feces is expelled painfully from the body. A liquid diet is essential in the initial phases of treatment. The liquid of choice is fat-free buttermilk or churned yogurt, but rice or oat milk often serves well for those who are intolerant of dairy. Buttermilk or yogurt soup, light miso broth, or rice gruel may also work well, spiced light-ly with ginger, garlic, fenugreek or black pepper (provided that the patient's Pitta is not already too disturbed). A similar diet must be continued until all the ama disappears from the stool, and the return to more solid food thereafter must be gradual.

When ama is profuse in the gut 1/4 tsp. two or three times a day of a mix-ture of one part ginger, two parts of cumin and three parts of haritaki, mixed into a paste with honey or molasses and licked slowly, can help dislodge it. Haritaki scrapes ama from the walls of the intestine, and ginger and cumin return tone and vitality to those walls.

Irritable bowel and colitis tend to develop when dysentery is neglected, when a fearful mind encounters persistently threatening situations that grip it in the pit of its figurative belly, or when both trends work together. In states of coli-tis Vata dries out and makes sticky the natural Kapha-produced mucus that lines the colon, which hinders healthy bowel motility. Characteristic symptoms include a griping pain and the passage of mucus in a series of unsatisfactory bowel movements that often leave the sufferer as feeling that he has passed nothing at all.

Castor oil, one ounce of more, taken internally with tea of powdered ginger, is often a good way to begin the job of stripping old adherent mucus from the colon's walls. The diet should be liquid here as well, for when the bowel is exceptionally irritated any "piece" of food may scrape it back into vexation. Retention enemas of oil can be used daily for several days until the colon again feels itself to be well-lubricated.

Treatment for cantankerous bowel is incomplete until one addresses the men-tal imbalances that facilitated its development. The most important of all medica-ments for the mind which controls a cantankerous bowel is calm and relaxation. When the mind acknowledges that it has pushed the bowel too far, and creates within the abdomen that vital space in which bowel health thrives, the gut will heal itself. Deep, slow, regular abdominal breathing is the one key building block for this vital space.

We must also address the consciousness of the intestine itself. We are able to consider these many intestinal conditions under the umbrella designation "cantankerous bowel syndrome" because bowels like other body parts have awarenesses of their own. These sensibilities are no doubt rudimentary, but they are influential nonetheless. A bowel goes surly when the mind and mouth stubbornly insult its intelligence with food of improper quality consumed in indefensible quantities at inadvisable moments again and again. Once grouchy, a bowel requires gentle personal attention to calm it down and induce it to return to its normal functioning. Only when it is again treated as a valued member of the body-mind-spirit family is a cantankerous bowel likely to resume its normal functions.

Asthma

Among the ailments that can be prevented by pacifying a cantankerous bowel is bronchial asthma. Bronchial asthma is usually spoken of as being "born from the stomach," and when Kapha or ama is its primary cause this is often literally true. But an uncooperative colon may so obstruct the normally downward-moving force of Vata therein that it may no longer be able to descend. When Vata's progress is thwarted in one direction it will usually seek to travel in the direction opposite, and indeed a Vata which can no longer travel down and out of the large intestine will usually choose instead to rise through the gut into the chest. There it will encourage shallow, unsatisfactory breathing, which can when conditions are right evolve into asthma.

Strongly Vata-aggravating emotions (fear, anxiety and grief in particular) can foment asthma on their own, even in the absence of significant Kapha or Ama, if they should find themselves being stored in the colon. These emotions are amplified significantly in the presence of overexertion and other Vata-enhancing factors, including particularly the habitual restraint of the body's natural urges. The thirteen natural urges which must never be restrained are the urges to: urinate, defecate, fart, vomit, sneeze, belch, yawn, ejaculate semen when aroused, eat when hungry, drink when thirsty, sleep when tired, pant when exhausted, and cry when miserable. Once exertion or urge-restraint or some other agent has ruffled Vata's feathers and caused it to move inappropriately upwards, the misplaced Vata can both create acute respiratory distress and can, by dispiriting the digestive fire, promote the production of ama, which will encourage that distress to become chronic.

However, it is far more common in the causation of asthma for Vata to have the help of pre-existing ama. Fatty, heavy, sticky, chilled or frozen or otherwise Kapha-producing food promotes asthma; dairy products are often among the worst offenders. Allergic or sensitivity reactions to food, dust, mold or pollutants compound the problem. Even climate can be implicated, for thunderstorms can sometimes trigger asthma attacks, even in people who have never before had one. Is it the pollen the winds stir up that does the dirty work, or the changes in barometric pressure or ion concentrations—or is it simply the production of a "storm" in the Vata of an internal cosmos which is resonating to an external storm?

Asthma is common during childhood, that period of life when Kapha is as constitutionally predominant in an individual as it will ever be. Fortunately, most cases of childhood asthma do not persist into adulthood. Some of the risk factors for adult asthma include a history of childhood asthma or of eczema (which is often ama-mediated) at any age; a parent who had a history of asthma; life in an urban environment, particularly one shared with pets, cockroaches, dust mites and molds; and being female. The age at which a woman has her first child may also be a significant factor.

Time of day also plays its part. Bronchial asthma is called in Sanskrit *tamaka shvasa* ("dark dyspnea") because, says an ancient text, "it always worsens at night." After the sun sets patients often feel that they are drowning in the ocean of night, oppressed by a feeling of inability to imbibe sufficient Prana from the atmosphere. The fact that Kapha predominates in the hours after sunset makes the situation worse. The physical fatigue of the day makes it more difficult to focus one's healing energies on oneself, and the fear that this sensation generates amplifies the distress. Even posture exerts an influence, for spasms are characteristically less while sitting and worse when lying down.

Chronic Kapha aggravation being, however, the most consequential of asthma's causes, treatment usually focuses on removing Kapha and ama and regulating Vata. Because asthma is a disease of "attacks" we can classify treatments for asthma according to whether they are used during or in between assaults.

During an attack the physician must first decide, by evaluating the strength of the patient relative to the disease's power, whether it is more appropriate to try to actively purify, or merely to pacify, the Doshas. An emetic effect (such as can often be obtained merely by filling the belly with licorice tea) is often the optimal purification for asthma in which Kapha is extreme. If instead Vata in the colon seems to be the main cause of the condition the best answer to the problem may be to administer an enema. This will remove whatever is preventing Vata from descending, thereby relieving pressure on the lungs. Moreover, when the large intestine works more efficiently it collects more Prana from the food ingested, which requires the body to take less Prana from ingested air, which provides the lungs with some rest.

When purification is not indicated, two ounces of strong licorice tea can be given with one ounce of medicated oil (such as Narayana Oil or Bala Oil) sipwise by mouth with simultaneous fomentation of the chest. The texts advise that "even those who should not be sweated (such as pregnant women) should be fomented, if only for a moment." Inhalation of the smoke of powdered datura (jimsonweed, locoweed) will cut short most any asthma attack.

Between attacks treatment will depend on the pattern and intensity of the dosha disturbance. Regular supervised practice of yoga postures and breathing is essential. Mineral medicines like Lakshmi Vilasa Rasa are particularly effective at preventing recurrences. Useful herbal compounds include the powders called Trikatu, Sitopaladi and Talisadi, the asafetida-containing preparation known as Hingvashtaka, jams like Chyvana Prasha and Agastya Haritaki, and medicinal wines containing long pepper, datura and ephedra.

All causative factors must be avoided, and food should be liberally spiced with ginger, garlic and turmeric to promote strength in the digestive fire and discourage the production of ama. When Vata gets unkinked and ama gets discharged the body will right itself, but the malady can always return so long as the stomach remains befouled and the bowel cantankerous.

The Yellow Peril

Even if a bowel be cantankerous, the toxins it dispatches into the system can still be discharged with a minimum of disquiet so long as that system's liver remains on its best behavior. One of the liver's chief tasks is to purify the blood, but even that hard-working organ's resolve can weaken when too many toxins assail it for too long.

The liver works with the spleen to keep the organism's blood healthy, and blood gradually loses many of its healthy characteristics as levels of toxicity rise. One of blood's cardinal attributes is its redness, and as it becomes polluted blood loses its healthy red hue, and becomes pale (as in anemia and leukemia). One's blood can be "pale" without being frankly anemic, for standard tests disclose quantities in blood, not its qualities. Blood may remain thus "pale" for years at a time.

When such a patient of "pale blood" strongly stimulates Pitta through his diet and activities his blood's pallor may take on a yellow (jaundiced) tinge. The liver is a predominantly Pitta-type organ, a yellow organ, and when Pitta rises so does the liver's yellowness. This yellowness may remain implicit in the blood until the individual comes into contact with a catalyst that galvanizes it to become explicit. Should the catalyst be exposure to a hepatitis virus, the yellowness may express itself in the form of a case of infective hepatitis.

Ayurveda groups infective hepatitis with all other conditions in which bile leaves its normal home in the liver and gall bladder and calls them as a group *kamala*. Kamala yellows the body's other tissues (particularly urine, feces, eyes, nails and skin), weakens the body and senses, produces burning sensations, and disrupts digestion. Other symptoms may include nausea and vomiting, giddiness, itching, excessive thirst or sweat, and loose stools. Kamala also create's changes in the mind's color, for it incites its victims to "see things with a jaundiced eye." Above all, the patient of Kamala lacks all desire in life, especially the desire for food; in Sanskrit the word kamala means "lack of desire."

It is only fitting that those afflicted by kamala should lack desire, for all too often their conditions developed from overabundance of desire. Yellowness enters regions of the organism where it does not belong thanks primarily to aggravation of Pitta, and overindulgence in substances and actions that stimulate desire is what primarily aggravates Pitta. Kamala is a special case of a more general disease that is called in Sanskrit *raga*. Raga, which also means "inflammation," "redness," and "musical mode," indicates in this context both "craving" and "surge." Pitta enhances appetites, and as an individual becomes Pitta-provoked the craving to surge forth in life becomes an itch that demands to be scratched.

Since Pitta facilitates indulgence in speed and intensity, the afflicted individual will crave to indulge in Pitta-arousing stimuli. Hot, spicy, sour, salty, fatty foods, oils, alcohol and flesh foods all enhance Pitta, particularly when they can act in concert with internal passion (*raga*) and external heat. Epidemiological studies suggest that the closer you live to the equator (and so, usually, the hotter your climate) the more likely you will be to suffer from liver diseases like hepatitis. And all these causative factors are much more likely to result in kamala when they appear in a person who is distressed by intense states of lust, jealousy, longing or wrath.

These causative factors combine to increase Pitta, which weakens the digestive fire's of body and mind, which facilitates the production of ama, which obstructs the free movement of gross and subtle substances in the body's various gross and subtle channels. This obstruction leads to Vata *prakopa* (provocation), which is magnified significantly by Pitta's innately provocative nature. Provoked Vata perverts the body's normal "space"; in such Pitta-toxic circumstances Vata will preferentially perturb organs and tissues like the liver which being high-Pitta themselves have already been weakened by Pitta excess. This aggravates Pitta all the more, and once it becomes sufficiently irate it climbs aboard Vata and takes off for a tour of all the tissues.

Prakopa literally means "extreme anger," which is the sort of emotional upset that is created in the cells of those tissues by the petulant Pitta and Vata. Even though each cell possesses a fairly minimal ability to express on its own, the accumulated roar of billions of incensed cells sends a surge of "extreme anger" to the brain, which can further unbalance the mind.

Once the liver has been badly "burned" by Pitta it may unhinge even the foundations of thought. Someone who suffers from a severe case of cirrhosis of the liver can go into a coma if he or she eats as little as one ounce of red meat, since the liver can no longer filter out all the false neurotransmitters produced during the meat's digestion. While a high protein diet will not cause those people whose livers are functioning subpar to lose consciousness, it is likely to distort their thinking and feeling.

The French have long recognized as a syndrome the "liver crisis" (*crise de foie*), a state of "yellow peril" brought on by overindulgence in rich foods and alcohol which requires to be rectified by a spell of purification, preferably at a well-appointed spa. *Crise de foie* can also be rendered *crise de foi* ("crisis of faith"), which is only to be expected when Vata and Pitta have addled one's body, mind and emotions. It is said that one reason why Napoleon failed at Waterloo was that he found himself in the midst of a crisis of liver/faith there, and could not take the time to take the cure.

Mellowing the Yellow

Whenever possible a deranged dosha should be brought back into balance while it is still accumulating in its home organ. "Pale" blood should thus be returned to robust redness before it gets the chance to become perilously yellow. Removal of the causative factors is both the ultimate remedy and the initial step. Diet and lifestyle must change, which will require that the mind relinquish that attitude of allurement that made overstimulation appear so attractive in the first place.

If liver disease has already developed, removal of the causes must be augmented by active therapeutic intervention. When the patient is relatively strong and the disease relatively weak, the physician should assist Nature in Her healing work by administering active purification. Jaundice may be due either to excess Pitta or to obstruction to Pitta's free flow. Excess-Pitta jaundice usually shows itself in the stools, which are often a fluorescent-yellow with bile. Such a condition calls for mild purification with Bitter substances.

When the patient's stools resemble in color and texture that paste of sesame seeds known as tahini an obstruction to the free movement of bile is likely, one that may be due to Vata, to Kapha, or to both. While Vata-caused impediments should generally be treated gently, Kapha-generated roadblocks are best remedied by careful administration of Pungent, Salty, very Sour, intense, hot, oily substances that will forcibly remove the obstruction. Either way, once the normal color of stool returns the Bitter regimen should be resumed.

Note that Pungent, Salty, very Sour, intense, hot, oily substances are what make up the "liver flush" that modern naturopaths administer to their patients of "liver crisis." A common recipe for a liver flush includes olive oil, ginger or garlic or cayenne (Pungent), and lemon juice (Sour). Such therapy can be very useful when given to the right patients, and when it is given only so long as the obstruction (be it structural or functional) remains. If liver flush therapy is continued after the blockage has been removed it will serve to stimulate the body to produce more bile, and more Pitta, which may in the long run make matters worse.

The same sort of diet that profits those who have abused alcohol works well with those whose livers have been damaged by other causes. Though the liver can regenerate even after severe damage, it is never quite the same as it was before being injured, and must be treated with some attention ever after. Bitter blood purifiers benefit people with active jaundice, those who are recovering from liver disease, and those whose livers have not yet been overwhelmed but are merely at risk. Some beneficial Bitter herbs are aloe vera, turmeric, dandelion, burdock, yellow dock, blessed thistle, gentian, barberry or Oregon grape, goldenseal, katuka, bhringaraja, punarnava and bhumyamalaki. It is usually advisable to change from one herb or mixture to another after a short period (one to three months), and to continue consuming such preparations in small, tonic quantities for months or years thereafter, delivering thereby a continuous mild stimulation that will keep the liver on its toes.

Preparations of iron like Punarnavadi Mandura or Mandura Vataka strengthen Blood as they scrape Pitta from the liver. Neem is especially good for the itching that often accompanies lever disease, but must not be used for too long in Vata-provoked people. A simple and effective recipe that alleviates jaundice involves mixing 1 tsp. of bicarbonate of soda with a few Tbsp. of fat-free yogurt (or better yet fresh buttermilk) taken internally twice daily.

No treatment for liver disease is complete without treatment of the mind that permitted yellowness to imperil the patient. A new, healthier self-image must be generated and inputted into the awareness, one that will promote faith, remind ahamkara of its limits, and discourage the sorts of surges that exhaust the system by "discoloring" and toxifying the blood.

Rheumatic Disease

Persistent toxicity facilitates the creation of enduring allergies that can eventually develop into more serious conditions. Ama becomes so tightly wedged into you that some of your own tissues are destroyed by immune reactions. Once dead these cells are themselves foreign bodies, ama from an internal source which the immune system engulfs and devours in the same way that it would attack intruders. Eventually your immune cells can acquire a cannibalistic taste for living tissue of the type that it has been scavenging. This is an "autoimmune" reaction.

Auto-immune disease has been described as conditioned, or limited, malignancy. Since auto-immune processes mediate the aging process, and since all of us die of old age if no other disease claims us earlier, autoimmunity must be eliminated before rejuvenation becomes possible.

Rheumatic disease provides a good example of an auto-immune condition that can often be successfully managed by an Ayurvedic approach. The rheumatic diseases—rheumatic fever, rheumatism, and rheumatoid arthritis—are conditions in which the body is filled with "rheum," a form of ama. About 10% of all patients who see a doctor have some rheumatic disease, an indication of how deeply ill the general public has become. Rheumatoid arthritis can, like rheumatic fever, affect the heart, and can actually kill. It is a serious, life-threatening condition.

Rheumatoid arthritis is a generalized systemic disease that can occur at any age, though it is less common in children and teenagers than it is in adults. Younger people are more prone to rheumatic fever, which is still common in some less developed countries and is basically an acute form of the same disease process. On average rheumatoid arthritis first appears around age forty. There is a hereditary tendency involved, and women are affected three to five times as often as men are. While it affects people in all parts of the world it is significantly more severe in cold, damp climates, which promote Kapha congestion and ama accumulation.

Rheumatoid arthritis is called in Sanskrit *Ama-Vata*, which means that it occurs when Vata circulates ama all throughout the body. The most important initiating cause seems to be improper diet, which creates ama. Other causes include exhaustion due to overwork, excessive exercise, frequent sex, intense worry, and emotional disturbances such as grief. Exhaustion and strong emotion make rheumatoid arthritis worse, and can sometimes initiate it, by aggravating Vata. Overuse of intoxicants, especially alcohol, simultaneously disturb Vata and create ama.

The sticky, opaque, offensive sludge that is ama can be found in the joints of every sufferer of rheumatoid arthritis. This is one sure way to distinguish rheumatoid arthritis from osteoarthritis, which is a localized manifestation of the aging process. When synovial fluid, that sticky, highly viscous lubricant which lubricates our joints, is withdrawn from an osteoarthritic joint it will be nearly normal. In rheumatoid or bacterial arthritis, however, the fluid loses its ability to lubricate, becomes turbid, contains cells of many types in large numbers, and even clots on standing. Healthy synovial fluid never clots.

Synovial fluid is one of the body's repositories of the force of Kapha. Kapha and ama are so alike in quality that it is not surprising that ama should have an affinity for the joints. Much of the ama that reaches the joints originates in the colon, where improper fat metabolism creates a variety of ama that shows a special affinity for the bones and joints. The membrane that lines the colon is intimately connected with the nutrition of cartilage and bone, and ama absorbed across this membrane will swiftly reach its preferred location and deposit itself. The immune system sweeps in to attack, and the disease is created. If allowed to continue unchecked the inflammation becomes chronic and destroys the joint, which causes nearby muscles to atrophy. All this transpires thanks to undigested material in the colon.

Menstrual irregularities predispose women to rheumatoid arthritis. Women are physically more fortunate then men in that each month their Blood is purified by the menstrual flow. During the first part of the month the body provides the womb the best possible nutrients to prepare it to host a child. If pregnancy does not occur the endometrium becomes superfluous and is transformed from essential tissues into ama, a foreign body that the womb must expel. The body takes advantage of this process to append to the menstrual flow all the filth that collected in Blood over the month. Even if a woman's digestion is not optimal in her gut she gets a second chance to nourish her higher dhatus properly by this monthly Blood purification. This is probably one reason that women live longer than men do.

Unfortunately this is a blessing only as long as the menses is regular and adequate. If for some reason a woman's menstrual flow is obstructed, and all filth is not eliminated from Blood, this virulent ama can perfuse her body and enhances the effects of other ama. Yogis maintain that one sign of spiritual advancement in a woman may be the natural cessation of menses, but this should happen spontaneously once the system has become thoroughly purified. Spiritual practices that teach women to suppress their menstruation are highly pernicious. Premature deliberate cessation of menstruation is fraught with perils including the possibility for the production of dangerous blood clots.

Emotion is a significant causative factor of arthritis. When you are upset, oppressed by grief, insecurity, fear or some other powerful emotion, you cannot pay proper attention to what or when you eat. You may throw yourself into your work or your play for that emptiness of mind that comes with exhaustion, or you may turn to intoxicants to escape the oppression of your misery. You know how your appetite evaporates when you are angry or otherwise upset. Food eaten when you have no appetite creates ama and acts as an insidious poison whose effects surface only gradually.

Unstable emotion can cause damage by making the mind seek escape from its condition through obsessive activity. It also affects the organism directly, as for example after an emotionally charged sporting event, when the rheumatic factor temporarily increases in the blood of affected players. Long-term unsettled emotion also seems to have an effect; rheumatoid arthritis is three times more common in individuals who were adopted as children than in those who lived with their genetic parents.

In psychotic arthritics symptoms of arthritis alternate with symptoms of psychosis, indicating that arthritis is one means that the organism uses to manifest severe mental distress without totally disrupting its balance of mind. The principal result of arthritis is severe crippling which prevents the patient from living a normal life, and in this it is very much like catatonia. Catatonics cannot move for psychological reasons. Arthritis sufferers have physical reasons for their immobility, and physical disability is much more socially acceptable than is mental disorder.

Arthritis sufferers are often psychologically rigid and inflexible. Suppose you are engaged in work you dislike, or you resent your boss, or you find your working conditions intolerable. If you will neither adapt nor admit to yourself your inability to adapt an attack of arthritis can give you a valid excuse to disengage yourself from work without any blame, since physical disease is supposedly "beyond your control."

Any intolerable role can result in physical stiffness that prevents or limits the necessity to play that role. Perhaps women are more prone to rheumatoid arthritis than are men, despite the fact that female sex hormones help alleviate the disease, because of ahamkara's confusion in determining their place in life. A woman who resents having to be submissive to her husband, or who despises the dependent role her society foists on her, is pulled in two directions. Drawn by two desires, for individuality and for union with her family and society, she is impaled on the horns of a dilemma. A physical condition helps her retain her fantasies of how she would live her life if she were free of restraint, without forcing her to act on those dreams. She knows inside how she wants to be, but may lack the courage and self-confidence to hurdle the barriers to her self-expression.

Insufficient strength to resist the influences that seek to fetter her indicates weakness of Bone, the dhatu that permits ahamkara to project herself into the world. Weakness of Marrow, which governs the joints, makes ahamkara fear failure every time she considers asserting herself. Fear of failure to self-assert combines with fear of the consequences of self-assertion to immobilize her. This disturbs Vata, creates Astringency, constricts her circulation, and promotes congestion. Her frustration continues to increase, magnifying the Bitterness in her being and further aggravating Vata, until finally the congestion of ama in the joint flares into inflammation and her arthritis manifests.

The disease is an actual entity, an alien servant she has created out of her ama to work for her. Now she need no longer slave away at household chores that go unappreciated by her family; she has altered her internal reality so that she need not adapt to external reality. For some sufferers rheumatoid arthritis becomes reality, security and sanity. They almost feel that they would disintegrate, that their identities would dissolve, if they relaxed, felt, wept, and returned to face external reality.

The disease is also an addiction, a crutch that makes it possible to cope. Unfortunately it is a very poisonous crutch. Ama eventually spreads to the heart, blood vessels, eyes, lungs, and nerves, resulting in anemia, swollen lymph nodes and increased heart rate. The heart complications sometimes prove fatal. Colitis, constipation, erratic blood pressure, bronchitis, kidney stones, leg cramps, and gall bladder disease can all develop as a direct result of rheumatoid arthritis. In severe cases amyloid, a type of internal ama that can cause death by clogging the kidneys, may get deposited.

Nowadays most sufferers from rheumatoid arthritis cannot pinpoint the day on which their disease began, for they suppress all symptoms as they arise. The pain and stiffness in their muscles and joints increase gradually over weeks or months accompanied by unusual tiredness and a general feeling of unease. In about one out of every ten victims, however, it still develops suddenly, following the descriptions of centuries-old Ayurvedic texts, with fever, severe malaise, body ache, indigestion, thickly furred tongue and loss of ability to taste in the mouth. The principal pathology involves swelling, redness and tenderness in one or several of the large joints. Typically the inflammation moves from joint to joint, dying back in one as it springs up in another, a symptom known as "wandering pain" in Sanskrit.

In some patients emotional causes outweigh physical influences; in others, physical causes predominate. Whatever the causation, physical medicine to expel ama from the body is essential in management of rheumatic disease because "rheum" is central to it.

Management of Arthritis

Arthritis of various types has afflicted vertebrates for a long, long time. At least since the time of the dinosaurs, in fact, according to the fossil record. Managing inflamed joints has become easier since those days, but is still not easy; it requires slow, patient attention, and an awareness that periods of improvement are likely to be punctuated by sudden, often unpredicted flare-ups. This can seem daunting at times; Sir William Osler, the justly famous Canadian physician, once said, "When a patient of arthritis walks in the front door, I feel like leaving out the back door."

But with patience progress can be and is made. Probably the first step to take in controlling a set of rheumatic joints is to acknowledge that your body may be being made to undergo conflict to protect your mind from having to confront confused or repressed feelings. If you can admit to yourself that you may have such an internal conflict and express to yourself the willingness to eventually deal with it you have taken the first step toward cure. Then you can use physical therapies to control the physical effects of the disease, confident that the hidden causes of your condition will not aggravate it while the physical housecleaning is going on.

You may find that this willingness to face reality, when combined with proper physical measures, is sufficient to control your disease, particularly if your disease was mainly due to improper diet and was only secondarily due to emotional causes. Even if your emotions were the primary cause, success with your joints will increase your confidence about the possibilities for healing, making it easier to deal with your mind later when you feel ready to do so.

Chronic rheumatoid arthritis like other auto-immune diseases displays two separate, alternating phases: exacerbation and remission. During the exacerbation phase all the typical symptoms are present and the joints are acutely inflamed. During remission the symptoms disappear as the acute accumulation of doshas in the joints dissipates. The doshas are still there at the joint, threatening mayhem; their threats are temporarily empty because they have become reduced lower than the threshold level necessary to manifest the disease. When a bucket under a tap becomes full it overflows. If you turn off the tap the bucket stops overflowing, but it is still full. As soon as the tap goes on again, even a trickle, the bucket will overflow once more.

Because there is such deep ama in arthritic joints any dosha accumulation in the digestive tract always tends to return to the joints and exacerbate the condition again. Health can return to the joint only after its bucket of ama is emptied. Effective management of arthritis involves immediate elimination of doshas during exacerbation, and gradual elimination of deep ama during remission. The basic philosophy of therapy for rheumatoid arthritis in summarized in a pithy Sanskrit saying:

**Fasting, sweating, and the Bitter and Pungent Tastes,
All to enkindle the digestive fire.**

EXACERBATION

Fasting – Food during an exacerbation should be *light, little,* and *liquid,* in the words of Dr. Vasant Lad. Weak ginger tea sipwise, with lemon and honey if necessary, is best when your tongue is thickly coated. Proceed gradually to rice or barley gruel, then thin mung bean soup, and finally to mung kichadi. Remain there until you go into remission, and at least a week longer, before you begin to return to your normal food. Remove all animal fats, even ghee, from your diet for two to six weeks.

You are probably allergic to several of the foods you commonly eat. After your digestion and appetite have improved, introduce only two or three of the foods you normally eat back into your diet each day, one at each meal, and examine yourself for reactions, like a sudden return of pain to the joint. If you are unsure about a reaction take your pulse both before and after eating. If your pulse increases 5% or more after your meal you are probably reacting to something that you ate. Anytime you have a reaction eliminate that food from your diet, and test it again after a week. If you still react to it give it up for at least six months before you try it again.

Regardless of your allergies, you should eliminate all animal fats, all fried foods, all dairy products, all refrigerator cold food, all white sugar, all alcohol, and all nightshades from your diet for at least six weeks, and preferably longer. The nightshades include potato, tomato, eggplant, peppers and tobacco. If you cannot give tobacco up entirely, restrict yourself as much as you can. If chilies form an important part of your diet they may have caused part of the problem, and you should eliminate them during this regimen. Curtail your use of salt. Drink your water hot.

Eliminate aluminum from your food. Aluminum is Astringent, which is why it is used in antiperspirants. It constricts body membranes and encourages ama to dry on them, making the ama more difficult to remove. The aluminium in antiperspirants is probably more bioavailable than that in other sources, but take no chances. Give away your aluminum cookware, and check to make sure that your baking powder is not aluminum-based.

Sweating – Wet heat aggravates obstruction and congestion; dry heat is more advantageous. A hot water bag or electric heating pad is one option. Another, better one is to heat in the oven a tray filled with brick dust, or with a mixture of equal parts of sand and powdered rock salt. Pour the heated powder into a cotton or linen bag and apply it to the joint. The dryness of these materials helps dry out the congestion in the joint. Applying oil to the joint before heating it will multiply the soothing effect, but since Vata is obstructed by ama, ordinary oil will increase the obstruction. Castor oil alone can reduce the inflammation and scrape out the ama, so apply a film of castor oil to the affected joint before applying heat. Sunbathing is doubly good for arthritic joints: the infrared rays provide healing heat, and the ultraviolet rays produce the vitamin D that is vital for the health of colon and Bone.

Poultices can also make the joint "sweat" by permeating it with the innate "heat" of the herbs used. Jimsonweed leaf (*Datura* species, known as stramonium or angel's trumpet in some areas) is a good, easily available material which is however poisonous and must be used with care. Its leaf can be crushed and bound over the joint with cloth, or a whole leaf can be coated with castor oil and applied after gentle roasting in a cast-iron pan. A thick paste of rhubarb root left to dry on the joint can help reduce its swelling. A paste of dry ginger helps the body digest the ama deep in the joint (don't leave it on so long that you burn your skin!). Comfrey root plasters soothe and heal, as do slippery elm and mullein. Lobelia, pine needles, and even cayenne are all appropriate in certain circumstances. Cayenne and nettles can also be used, except by Pitta people or in intense inflammation, to irritate the joint into beginning to purify itself.

Bitter and Pungent – These tastes are used to help control Vata and relieve ama. In general, because Pungent is Hot in Energy it is best to use Pungent substances during remission to actively rekindle the digestive fire. Bitter substances are better during exacerbation; they rekindle digestion indirectly and help reduce inflammation. Bitter is especially needed when there is severe and generalized body ache, loss of appetite, lack of taste in the mouth, indigestion, and fever.

Fever is the body's way of sending heat to the dhatus to help digest ama. Even modern medicine has finally realized that fever is an important mechanism for destroying pathological microbes and viruses. Fever should be suppressed, with cold compresses, only if it climbs too high, usually above 101°F. Bitter substances catalyze fever's digestive action on ama and permit the fever to finish work and subside sooner.

Some commonly available substances which are wholly or partly Bitter include:

Alfalfa	Chicory	Licorice Root
Aloe Vera	Dandelion	Red Clover
Barbérry	Devil's Claw	Skullcap
Birch	Echinacea	Yarrow
Burdock	Gentian	Yellow Dock
Chickweed	Golden Seal	Yucca

While all Bitter substances can benefit arthritis at this stage, each possesses specific properties. Gentian is useful when there is significant loss of appetite along with indigestion. Aloe vera soothes the digestive tract and purifies the liver. Barberry and dandelion are both good liver purifiers. Alfalfa is a natural pain reliever and purifies the colon. Devil's claw and yucca help relieve joint pain. Licorice root exerts an anti-inflammatory effect. Skullcap soothes nerve irritation. Bayberry, echinacea and golden seal help eliminate parasitic microorganisms.

All Bitter substances help reduce the tendency to allergy by toning and rebalancing the metabolism. Ayurvedic compounds like Tikta or Mahasudarshan Churna, both of which are extremely Bitter, actively help eliminate the allergic state from your system if used regularly for at least six weeks. Such substances can also interrupt or prevent certain allergic reactions.

Guggulu is the substance of choice to control inflammation in rheumatoid arthritis. It is mainly Bitter in Taste, though its secondary Tastes are Pungent, Astringent and Sweet. Its Energy is Hot and its Post-Digestive Effect is Pungent. Triphala Guggulu is often useful in such conditions, since Triphala purifies the system and Trikatu improves its digestion.

The best compound of guggulu to use in an exacerbation of rheumatoid arthritis is, however, Simhanada Guggulu. It contains Makshika Bhasma, Triphala,

Sulfur, guggulu and castor oil, all prepared together in an iron pot. Makshika Bhasma is incinerated pyrite, which contains iron and sulfur. Iron scrapes ama from the tissues; sulfur purifies Blood. Guggulu scrapes ama from the joints, exerts an anti-inflammatory effect, and improves metabolism of Fat. All these substances are rejuvenators.

Castor oil is a specific for rheumatoid conditions. The word *simhanada* means "lion's roar," and as a Sanskrit verse comments:

> *The lion of castor oil alone can kill the maddened elephant of*
> *rheumatic disease as it stampedes through the body.*

Castor oil increases digestion by controlling Vata and scraping ama from colon and Bone. If the digestive tract is coated with ama it is wise to begin therapy by giving 2 to 4 Tbsp. of castor oil plus a cup of strong tea of dry ginger to thoroughly flush the colon and give a head start to purification of the joints.

Castor oil is Pungent, as is sulfur and, to some extent, guggulu. Pungent items can readily be used even in an exacerbation if there is much ama that needs to be eliminated and if there is no intense inflammation or other symptom of great involvement of Pitta. P people, except when full of ama, must be wary of most Pungent substances.

Common Pungent herbs include:

Basil	Garlic	Peppermint
Calamus Root	Ginger	Spearmint
Catnip	Lobelia	Turmeric
Fennel	Mugwort	Valerian
Fenugreek	Parsley	Wood Betony

Although Pungent, the mints generally do not increase Pitta unless they are used in excess. This is also the case for turmeric.

One simple recipe for rheumatic complaints, especially those involving only one joint, is to grind a clove of garlic in a tablespoon of milk and consume it just before bedtime. Although dairy products are specifically forbidden in this condition, this tiny amount of milk acts as a vehicle for the garlic and reduces its hot, irritating qualities.

In extreme inflammation, when Pitta is exceedingly increased, it is better to use Kaishora Guggulu, a form of guggulu prepared with the herb guduchi, which reduces guggulu's Hot and Pungent qualities.

REMISSION

Eating a balanced, anti-allergenic diet is the sort of fasting appropriate when the exacerbation diminishes. Wet heat can be used. Good Ayurvedic oils for rheumatic conditions are Dhanwantram Taila, Ksheerabala Taila, Sahachara Taila, Pinda Taila and Vishagarbha Taila. Vishagarbha Taila, which is poisonous, is useful even during an exacerbation. All these oils are medicated to purify and lubricate the joint. Occasional medicated enemas, especially when bowel habits change and the lower tract is full of gas, are useful to keep Vata under control and to encourage the lining of the colon to keep clearing itself of ama.

Guggulu is useful during remission to remove old, adherent ama from the dhatus. The best varieties here are Yogaraja Guggulu and Mahayogaraja Guggulu. Both contain more than two dozen Pungent herbs for improving digestion, and Mahayogaraja also contains minerals, for a greater rejuvenating effect.

During exacerbation it is sometimes necessary to stay in bed until the joint inflammation dies down. Moving an inflamed joint too vigorously may damage it further and may push the ama deeper into it. Once inflammation recedes, however, the joint must be kept mobile to minimize muscular atrophy and to circulate the synovial fluid within it. When this circulation is interrupted toxic ama has an opportunity to accumulate and induce fresh inflammation.

Simple Yoga postures and breathing exercises encourage elimination of ama. As your health improves supplement the Yoga with more energetic exercise, particularly in water, where your body weight is partially supported and the stress on your joints is correspondingly reduced. A regular exercise program is especially important for arthritis sufferers who are overweight since heavy limbs put extra strain on muscles and joints.

Some people notice that a pleasurable sexual experience temporarily removes arthritis pain. This results from a combination of psychological effect and release of pain-killing chemicals in the brain. While sex may occasionally be used for quick relief it is unwise to use sex as a painkiller habitually because excessive sexual activity weakens the nerves and exhausts ojas. Weak nerves and exhausted ojas will weaken digestion, increase ama, and worsen the arthritis. Do not pay for short-term relief with long-term misery.

Cortisone and other anti-inflammatory drugs like phenylbutazone are other common short-terms measures that may on occasion be necessary to prevent severe joint damage. They must not be used habitually, though, because they do not address the ama that is the cause of the condition. Drugs like cortisone are actually bribes to the immune system to induce it to look the other way while more ama is smuggled into the dhatus. If you are using corticosteroids regularly you must *never* stop them suddenly; this can be extremely dangerous. You must taper off from them very gradually under professional supervision.

Even "ordinary" pain relievers must be used with caution. One of every four people who use NSAIDs (non-steroidal anti-inflammatory drugs) for chronic pain develop ulcers. Using antacids to control the ulcers doubles the risk of developing a bleeding ulcer. Bleeding ulcers caused by NSAIDs kill an estimated 10,000 to 20,000 people annually while hospitalizing ten times that number. We need as a society need to learn to tolerate some pain instead of searching for a pill that will remove it from us instantly. Pain tells us not to use that painful limb, perhaps because it requires rest. When you take painkillers indiscriminately you may reinjure the part, creating greater pain for yourself further down the line. Knowing when to rest (to calm Vata) and when to be active (to stimulate Kapha and dispel ama) is one of the great challenges of rheumatic disease.

Meditation that helps people separate their thoughts and emotions from their physical sensations has been shown to dramatically reduce pain and improve mood in people with chronic pain.

Once in remission you should deal with your emotional conflicts. Perhaps the situation that aggravated you existed at one time but no longer exists now. Perhaps the cause of your disease was a past experience and your suffering is its delayed effect. If you look into yourself and find no deep confusion it may never have existed, or it may have disappeared after creating in you the alien being which now ravages you.

If you do locate an emotional maelstrom you must examine it without prejudice. The Bitter Taste in your supplements will help you admit your dissatisfaction to yourself. There is no benefit in assigning blame for that dissatisfaction. Dealing with present reality is more important. If you are having difficulty being objective about your situation ask for help from a trusted friend or a professional counselor. Do not make a habit of emotional purgation lest it begin to intensify your misery, just as overuse of the Pungent Taste increases Pitta and therefore anger.

Do not empower the alien personality you have created for yourself by giving it more importance than it is worth. You created it to do a job for you, and it did its job. Now that you have no further need of it you can allow it to go. As ama departs and the dhatus return to health ahamkara will become stronger, and you will be able to find in your "self" the satisfaction you may not have been able to locate externally. Love and compassion for yourself are the strongest remedies that exist for any disease, and the best nourishment for your immune system.

Cancer

Love and compassion are even more important in malignancy, another disease in which an alien personality is created. In arthritis the entity, like a good slave, performs the function it was created for. In cancer the alien alter ego rebels and turns on its maker. Taking over a renegade cell, the rebel proliferates, creates a body for itself and challenges ahamkara to a cancerous civil war for possession of the organism. The moment that ahamkara gives in and admits that all is lost the cancer becomes terminal.

It seems amazing that ahamkara, who adores life and tries to stay alive as long as she possibly can, could surrender and relinquish her authority to a murderous upstart. Sometimes overwhelming physical pollution that makes the body uninhabitable, such as intense or long-term exposure to chemical carcinogens or to radiation, is the cause. Sometimes an individual whose digestion has been impaired for many years develops cancer because of ancient residual ama. And sometimes extreme hopelessness can so overwhelm ahamkara and the immune system that a cancer arises.

The power of hopelessness is such that even people who have well-integrated personalities may develop cancers if the shock of some loss is too intense. Even a temporary spell of hopelessness may be sufficient to initiate a cancerous chain of events in someone whose body is filled with life-long physical ama accumulation. And, substantial exposure to powerful chemical or radioactive carcinogens can engender hopelessness in the cells of the body, who sense the fatal implications of the exposure. This cellular hopelessness is eventually fatal to the personality.

Weakness of Blood, the dhatu that provides invigoration to ahamkara, is critical to cancer development. In fact hemolysis (destruction of the blood) is common in cancer. Here again Blood loses its proper "color." So long as Blood is red—full of healthy red cells—it nourishes and invigorates all the dhatus and provides them Prana. When instead Blood becomes "white"—filled with the white cells of the immune system, which shows that the system has shifted its emphasis from nutrition of the dhatus to elimination of ama and aliens—it can no longer provide proper invigoration. Lack of Prana, transported by oxygen, encourages the growth of cancerous tissue, which hates oxygen. "White Blood" encourages hopelessness at the cellular level.

A cancer often results when an individual undergoes a physical or mental experience that is utterly indigestible by the personality, something that the being cannot face under any circumstances. Ahamkara is so unwilling to face the reality she isolates it, and by that very act, she creates an identity and individuality to the indigestible fact. That forever-alien experience lies in wait in the organism until it finds an abnormal, rebellious cell in which to live, and an invader is born.

When this "individual" finds a suitable host cell it "possesses" it, as a disembodied spirit might possess a human being. Because the fact is unbearable to ahamkara it is categorized as disruptive or "evil" from the onset, so when it is let loose in the body it destroys, true to the role assigned it. Cancer is too often a self-fulfilling prophecy. Even the belief that "everyone else can get cancer, but not me," which is a sign of mental indigestion, often masks a strong subconscious fear or anticipation of that very event.

Cancer production usually involves many factors in varying degrees of influence. Common to all cancers, however, is the incubation of initiating substances (carcinogens) in damaged cells and the possession of these cells by a self-generated alien personality. Sometimes ama itself can act as a carcinogen. Even if it does not, ama is essential for cancer proliferation because it is undigested material. Undigested thought and undigested food naturally gravitate to one another and nourish one another. Cancer cells receive their physical nourishment from ama irrigation and their mental encouragement from hopelessness.

It has been reported that a majority of cancer patients were not breast-fed. This may deprive them of some essential immune substance carried in the breast milk, or it may deprive them of early bonding with their mothers, or both. Good bonding with others begins with a good maternal bond. Poor bonding with others usually affects ahamkara's ability to bind to the dhatus, and encourages alien cells to bind instead.

Lack of good quality human bonding plus awareness of this lack, at whatever level ahamkara permits it to surface, may together form a key. The retarded and the criminally insane are reported to develop cancer at only half the rate of "normal" people who share their physical circumstances. Moreover, since a substantial number of cancer-free people all over the world smoke and drink their ways merrily past one hundred years of age, it would seem that either satisfaction with or unawareness of your situation in life reduces your likelihood of developing a malignancy.

Potential cancer patients may feel early on a deep sense of existential loneliness in their lives, and may erect barriers to keep others from loving them. They tend to keep a smile plastered to their faces, and rarely complain about anything. They may give much more than they receive, and may feel uncomfortable about accepting anything from others. This Astringent constriction which inhibits Salty enjoyment causes inability to accept Sweet nourishment from others, and guarantees disappointment in relationships because the giving is so needy. The Bitterness of disappointment may create unfocused Pungent anger or Sour envy. Once all Tastes are sufficiently unbalanced ahamkara may decide that life is no longer worth living.

Many people with cancer share psychological traits with people who commit suicide. Some people use a gun, a noose or pills to end themselves when the last straw drops onto them; others commit psychic suicide, and withdraw from the world into schizophrenia. Cancer-prone people invite a malignant hit man into them when they are ready to give up the ghost. As they decline they may finally allow themselves to accept assistance, given permission to do so by the disease, which is supposedly not their fault.

Any powerful dissatisfaction can affect ahamkara. Cervical cancer most often strikes either women who are lifelong virgins or those who are extremely sexually promiscuous. The former shun a pleasure which they feel they do not deserve, the latter embrace the pleasure but ensure that they do not receive real fulfillment from it, which they are sure they do not deserve. Men who suffer from such sexual uncertainty are likewise more prone to prostate cancer.

Such emotionally cancer-prone individuals often find some external reason for living. A special risk for cancer exists in those people whose meaning in life comes entirely from outside themselves. They may live for their jobs, or their families, or their causes, noble or ignoble. Whatever they are living for they become addicted to, investing everything they have in that external crutch, empowering it totally. Loss of this investment is a crushing blow, for ahamkara then must quit her addiction cold turkey. Unless some substitute can be quickly found, terminal despair and final dejection may set in, and the stage is set for one of the estimated 100,000 cancer cells which arise each day in the body to establish its own regime.

These cells may begin in any dhatu, though when a cancer is unchecked it eventually eats through them all. Vata makes cancer cells abnormal, and makes them proliferate rapidly. Kapha provides the uncontrolled increase in cell mass, and Pitta is in charge of robbing nutrition from other dhatus to feed the interloper. Cancer is at once a tornado of Vata that disrupts normal bodily functions and structures, a raging forest fire of Pitta that consumes the dhatus, and a great tidal wave of Kapha whose flood inundates all dhatus with its ama-poison. The doshas, which preserve the body in peaceful times, destroy it when disease gains control of them.

Consumption

This disease category represents several terminal conditions, among them tuberculosis and AIDS. It is also called "emaciation," or "chronic wasting syndrome," descriptions that are regarded as diagnostic of AIDS infection in a virus carrier. Ayurveda calls it consumption because it occurs when a disease completely overruns an individual, "consuming" him or her. As in cancer all doshas, all dhatus and all Tastes are disturbed in this condition, which differs from cancer in that a consumptive's mindset is the precise opposite of a cancer patient's. Consumptives and cancer patients both have loneliness in common, but consumptives rarely doubt their self-worth. Usually they are sure that they deserve the enjoyments of life, and put their wishes and desires before those of anyone else. They take what they want, regardless of the result.

The chief cause of consumption is willfulness. Consumptive types think they can do anything, and terminally overstrain themselves in order to prove it. Here ahamkara is so overconcerned with sensory gratification that she indulges in repeated "crimes against wisdom" and neglects to properly nourish her body.

Consumption develops in one of two ways. Taking in more nutrients of any sort than you can digest, particularly by excessive indulgence in improper diet, fills the system up with ama and aggravates Kapha. Excessive indulgence in exercise or sex, excessive discipline like fanatic fasting and penance, or excessive use of tobacco, alcohol, drugs and other intoxicants exhaust Ojas, starve the dhatus and aggravate Vata. Continual restraint of any natural urge also disturbs Vata.

Common to all these causes is "too much." Ahamkara tries too hard to show off, to demonstrate that she is better, brighter, stronger, smarter, tougher, more talented and generally more valuable than anyone else in the world. In trying to exceed herself she succeeds only in exceeding her limitations.

Excessive nutrition causes Kapha and ama to block the pathways for dhatu nutrition and obstructs the proper movement of nutrients, which is controlled by Vata. Insufficient intake of nutrients to replace an excessive outflow of energy, especially from repetitive, unsatisfying sex, directly disturbs Vata, whose dry, light and rough qualities exhaust the dhatus. Both processes rob the dhatus of nourishment, decrease Ojas and weaken immunity, permitting parasitical beings to colonize the system. The problem is not tubercle bacilli, Candida yeast, the Epstein-Barr virus, or even the AIDS virus. The problem is immune weakness, which is due to aggravated Vata.

We Americans guard our commitment to excess as if to prove our individuality to ourselves. Our gas guzzlers must be bigger than anyone else's; our GNP must be most colossal. We enjoy and enjoy, with no thought for tomorrow or for anyone else's tomorrow. We organize our lives around bread and circuses. But we cannot forever expand our indulgences, any more than we can endlessly expand our economy, because the disease of consumption lies in wait for all who overconsume and attempt to aggrandize themselves at the expense of the rest of Nature's creation.

There is no single therapy for cancer and consumption. The Ayurvedic approach to both involves whittling away at the strength of the disease while rebuilding the individual's immune power, to create a climate in which Nature can cure. Whatever the therapy, rejuvenation is essential to invigorate the dhatus and revitalize the organism.

In potentially fatal diseases like cancer and consumption the normal sequence of treatment steps is reversed. When you are injured in an accident you must initially get first aid for the injury, and then worry about everything else. Likewise, in serious disease you may first have to preserve life and only then consider how to purify and balance the system.

Therefore, for cancer and consumption, our procedure often becomes:

Rejuvenation first,
to preserve life.

Balancing the doshas second,
to strengthen the patient and weaken the disease.

Panchakarma next,
to purify the system.

Removal of the emotional cause of the condition thereafter,
when the patient is ready for it.

This may hold true even if the disease is not yet grave, especially when a mental predisposition is the main cause. One of my friends complained that whenever the pressure to "achieve"—in her work, in her relationship—mounted in her it would eventually create a fever. The fever would burn away all her accumulated nervous energy and leave her temporarily relaxed, but would return again and again. She asked my advice.

I told her that a major portion of her difficulty was due to her insistence on trying to use her will force to solve her problems. When her boss complained or her boyfriend argued she would throw herself into the situation in an assault on the walls preventing free communication.

After reminding her that the only result you can expect from beating your head on a brick wall is a sore skull I suggested that she first *rejuvenate* herself with nourishing herbs and with her favorite activities, and put all else on hold when she felt the fever rising. Once the crisis passed, I suggested that she *balance* the energy of interaction with the boss or the boyfriend, and that only after calm had returned should she try to *purify* the relationship by *removing the cause* of the disagreement.

Other Conditions

Insistence on trying to impose your will on every detail of your life can lead to many more than just the above illnesses, of course. The so-called "chronic fatigue syndrome" is a good example of what happens when you try to do too many things for too long. One of the most difficult barriers for most sufferers from chronic fatigue to surmount is the barrier of limitation, the idea that they may no longer be able to rely on seemingly limitless reserves of energy. Their energy reserves never were limitless—had they been they would never have fallen sick—but they had been able to convince themselves that they were, until they crashed.

A majority of sufferers from chronic fatigue seem to be P people, the types who rarely take no for an answer until Nature forces them to do so. And like good Ps most of them continue to try to ignore "no" even after they have no energy to resist. As soon as a little energy returns to them they tend to grab hold of it and run with it, thinking they are "cured." When they crash again their frustration, and the P-mediated internal corrosion that it creates, mounts exponentially. Until they are ready to surrender the obstinacy that characterizes the intact P nature, successfully returning from chronic fatigue is very difficult for them.

Lupus is often a Pitta-predominant disease, another permutation of "do-it-all" syndrome. Like rheumatoid arthritis it proceeds in cycles of exacerbation and remission and, as with arthritis, guggulu is frequently beneficial, particularly Kaishora Guggulu. Punarnavadi Guggulu and Gokshuradi Guggulu are also often used, particularly to prevent or slow kidney involvement.

Multiple sclerosis (MS) is a complex condition that attacks the fatty myelin on certain nerves that govern voluntary movements. MS seems to have two main "varieties." One is a Kapha-mediated variety in which the most important causative factors are a cold, wet climate coupled with a diet high in animal fat. The other is a high-energy, "overdo everything" variety which mainly affects Vata and Pitta. In the one the nerves appear to become exha,usted after being damaged by excess ama, in the other the damage seems to come first and the ama follows afterward. Eventually the two processes merge, and symptoms of Vata aggravation begin to dominate.

Treatment of MS begins, as usual, with removal of the cause, which begins with identification of the cause. The cold wet variety requires that the body be acitvated and stimulated, while the high, dry variety require that the body be calmed and replenished. In both cases the inflammation must be brought under control. Guggulu compounds are also useful, but can do little on their own. Dietary changes and a healthy routine focusing on Vata-controlling practices are essential to potentize the guggulu. Regular, gentle Yoga is a must, as it is in most diseases that involve the musculoskeletal system, including fibromyalgia, which is yet another disease whose pathology combines emotional with physical exhaustion.

Again and again we return to stress, and to our faulty response to it. If you fail to relax and regroup when stress hits you, your imbalances will age you quickly; stress will *consume* you. Systematic rejuvenation is the best answer for the problem of the unnatural stresses of our modern lives.

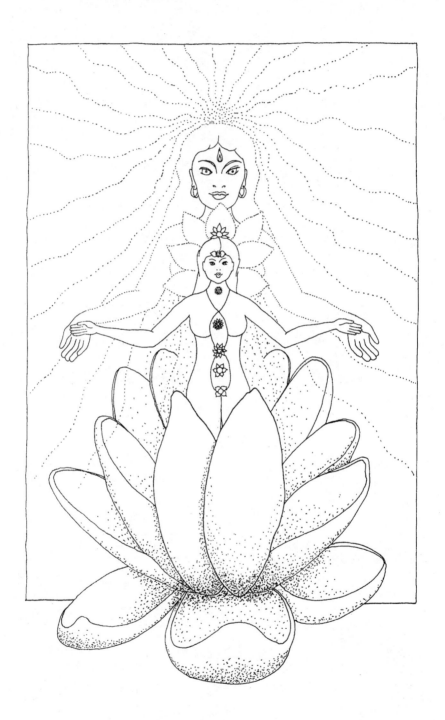

Chapter Eight
Rejuvenation

Disease always forces us to confront our attachments. All attachments are temporary and are dissolved by Nature when She feels it is time to broaden our personalities. Disease is always an opportunity to learn from our mistakes, an opportunity that Nature provides us out of Her maternal magnanimity. She hopes we will learn enough that we need never be sick. She can even teach us how to overcome death and to develop permanent personalities like the immortals. Rejuvenation is the first step in the direction of immortality.

Old age is an auto-immune disease, an admission by ahamkara that she is no longer adequately able to identify with the body. Old age is caused by repeated indulgence in sensory pleasures, whose wear and tear on the body destroys Ojas. The faster you live the faster you will deteriorate. Hummingbirds flit just a few seasons, but tortoises plod along for decades and centuries. Longevity requires slowness, for a slow life permits your protective aura to interpose itself more efficiently between you and the outside world.

The word used in Ayurveda for both rejuvenation and rejuvenating substance is *rasayana*, which literally means "the Path of Rasa." To walk the Path of Rasa you must purify and nourish your physical Rasa Dhatu, since Rasa is the raw material from which the other dhatus are formed. Healthy Rasa Dhatu is the first step in the physical production of healthy Shukra, from which Ojas is directly produced. Careful selection of food tastes (Rasas) and control of emotions (Rasas) ensures production of healthy Rasa Dhatu, which can then generate healthy Shukra and Ojas.

Because Shukra is best nourished by Sweet, rejuvenation requires creation of powerful Sweetness in body and mind. Honey is made of pollen, the sperm of plants. Plant Shukra increases human Shukra, according to the principle "like increases like." Honey is, therefore, innately rejuvenating. Honey is in addition a predigested food, thanks to those industrious bees, and it can enter any part of the body without having to be first digested. It can also do this for any medicine mixed with it, which is why it is valued as the best of all vehicles for therapeutic and rejuvenating substances. Mixing raw, unfiltered honey into your herbal tea allows honey to act as a vehicle for the active principles of the herb. Because honey is made poisonous by heating, however, it should be added after the tea is brewed and has cooled to the temperature at which you will drink it.

In honor of its position as the ideal Sweet food, honey is called *madhu* in Sanskrit. Madhu means "perfection of Sweet," in contrast to *madhura*, which refers to Sweet that must be first digested before it can give its Sweetness to ahamkara. All other physical substances are merely madhura; only honey is madhu.

Virilization

Most rejuvenators including honey are also aphrodisiacs, because both classes of substances increase Shukra Dhatu. A tremendous increase in Shukra usually inflames the fires of lust and causes a craving for sexual gratification. If you want a rejuvenating effect from a rejuvenating substance you must avoid arousal and contain the energy within you so that it can be digested into Ojas.

Onions increase Shukra quickly. But because they promote Rajas they make it more difficult for you to retain the Shukra long enough to convert it into Ojas. Onions produce Shukra but also cause the mind to search for a sexual situation in which to expend it. Ghee, the metal gold and mercury sulfide also produce Shukra quickly and also increase Rajas, though they and honey are less Rajas-producing than are onions.

Ayurveda separates the sciences of virilization and rejuvenation because virilization, besides increasing Shukra, also involves techniques for enhancing both sexual pleasure and fertility. Mutual pleasure is essential in sex; in fact, Charaka, Ayurveda's most eminent author, says that the best of all virilizers is a partner who loves you. Sex is more important to a woman than it is to a man, say the ancient texts. Modern medicine has in fact found that male pheromones, imbibed by a woman during the sex act, help regulate her fertility and ensure the health of her reproductive system. Regular sexual intercourse improves a woman's well-being.

Unsatisfactory sex is the cause of much disease in today's world, especially among women. A woman has every right to become angry if her man fails to satisfy her sexually, because he is withholding essential nutrients from her. Inadequate nutrition increases Vata, making her periods more erratic and difficult. Sexual frustration creates anger, and the Pungency created by anger imbalances a female's sexual organs and Blood and further affects her menstruation. Menstrual disturbances heighten a woman's emotional aggravation.

It is difficult for such a woman to become pregnant, and should she become pregnant her misery will be transferred to the child in her womb by the toxins circulating in her impure blood. Any baby grown in such a Bitter and Pungent environment will grow up dissatisfied and angry because those emotions are the foundation of that child's constitution.

Virilization is rejuvenation for Shukra Dhatu, and it is "pre-juvenation" for your children. Virilization is a method for selecting the healthiest possible genes a couple can muster to create a child with the healthiest possible constitution. This art of loving strengthens the male and female bodies and creates in them maximum excitement at the moment of congress. Some of that joy and excitement is transmitted into the zygote and provides a foundation of satisfaction on which the child can base its life.

Desire is the first disease, says the Ayurvedic writer Vagbhata. If a zygote can be infused with some of the immense satisfaction that a couple feels at the moment of orgasm, the child who develops will be more easily satisfied with life than a child whose parents copulated only for fun. And the child whose parents were convulsed by powerful, twisted emotions at the time of conception often ends up with constitutional hungers it can never quite satiate.

The foundation of sexual stress is loss of Ojas, which arises from sexual overindulgence. Many modern couples fail to take the time to properly enjoy sex, and seek only self-gratification instead of mutual satisfaction. Masturbation is the culmination of this tendency, the apex of self-indulgence and gratuitous waste of energy. The repetitive performance of unsatisfying sex is certain to cause disease.

Individuals lose the willingness to surrender themselves to each other in sexual union when they feel vulnerable because of weak identities. Lack of Ojas, due especially to frequent obsessive sex, weakens the aura, and whenever anyone gets too close subliminal alarm bells begin to go off. Every personality is organized differently, and the melding of auras that occurs when two people unite sexually is inherently threatening to ahamkara. If she has been weakened by weak Ojas she can feel overwhelmed by the opposing personality, sensing that her defenses are insufficient to protect herself. She may then paroxysmally thrust the partner away, physically or emotionally.

Many degrees of rejuvenation exist, but rejuvenation even to a minor degree is possible only when you discipline your sexual activity. Sex is the third Pillar of Life, and your attitude to sex must reflect its importance to your health. Reverence for sex is the real significance behind the philosophy of sexual restraint called *brahmacharya*, which literally means "that which brings you closer to the Creator." Yogis interpret this in a religious sense and follow the path of celibacy. Ayurveda interprets it to mean "that which causes the Creative Energy of the universe to accumulate within you."

Sex is the Pillar of Life most closely associated with Vata. Orgasmic sex is a tremendous energy drain on the system. Castrated salmon, for example, live twice as long as their potent counterparts simply because they do not exhaust themselves sexually. Sexual activity must always be carefully regulated lest it vitiate Vata.

It is best, for example, to enjoy sex at night, since night is ruled by Kapha, and Vata disturbance is less likely to result from sexual exertion then. Ayurveda suggests that orgasmic sex be limited to not more than twice a week in winter, when the body's internal fire is highest. In the spring and fall once a week is the suggested maximum frequency, and in summer, when the body is ravaged by heat, sex is indicated only once every two weeks. Yogis are even stricter, suggesting no more than once a month. Everyone should abstain from sex during illness and convalescence, and during menstruation.

Because the frequency of sexual activity should be limited to preserve physical health, and because unsatisfactory sex is an important cause of disease, the quality of each sexual experience must be enhanced. Meditation alone can do this. Sex itself should be made into a meditation, or an act of ritual worship, which can actually increase Ojas instead of decreasing it.

One of the *Upanishads* (spiritual treatises that explain the hidden meanings of the Vedas) describes all life in the cosmos in terms of sacrifice into fire. The world beyond is a form of the universal Fire, as is our world, and the gods send rain to transmit water from the one to the other. In the internal cosmos of the human body, the world beyond is the brain, the rain is the Ojas, and the gods are the mind and the senses. Our world is the physical body.

A human body is also a fire. Its open mouth is the fuel, its breath the smoke, its speech the flame, its eyes the coals, its ears the sparks. Into this fire, which represents the digestive processes in the dhatus, the gods offer food; from this offering arises Shukra. A woman's body has a special fire, a sexual fire. During intercourse the penis is the fuel, the pubic hairs the smoke, the vulva the flame, penetration the coals, and pleasure the sparks. Into this fire the gods offer semen. From this offering arises a new human being.

Two people performing sex should sacrifice all restraint, all doubts and uncertainties which separate them from each other and prevent them from becoming one, into the momentary unity experience of orgasm. Until you can convert your sexual experiences into meditations you will always be tempted to search for new sexual partners to satisfy your appetites, never able to locate that total sense of satisfaction which ordinary sex hints at but cannot achieve.

Successful sexual satisfaction occurs between two partners, not between two genital organs. It does not happen immediately, but grows and develops over time. The first step in improving your sexual experience is to resist the temptation to hop from bed to bed to seek improved pleasure. Stick to one partner, at least for a substantial period of time. V people are tempted by variety more than are other types; they should satisfy this craving for variation with new techniques and positions, not with new partners.

P people also have roving eyes, but their principal urge is for intensity of experience, and not variation. They have to be careful not to completely dominate a weaker partner, or worse, to permit their craving for intensity to mesmerize them into perversion. K people are least likely to roam, and since sex is a good vigorous exercise for them they can be encouraged to enjoy it more often than Ps or Vs, for whom ordinary sex is more a luxury than it is for Ks.

The first step in any virilization program is absolute sexual chastity for a month or more. It takes at least a month for the body to rebuild its Ojas stores so that ahamkara can feel sufficiently secure within herself to permit another being to come into intimate contact with her. Selective chastity, the practice of observing physical continence while actively fantasizing about sex, is useless. Sex is all in the brain anyway; no excitement occurs unless the mind wills it to occur. The continuous pressure of unresolved sexual thoughts is more detrimental to Ojas than is the physical loss of Ojas during the sex act. Moreover, the mental duplicity and deception involved leads to deviousness, which promotes willfulness and encourages other diseases to develop.

As with rejuvenation, full purification must precede virilization. Thereafter medicated oils should be applied regularly to the genitals to nourish and invigorate them. Internally, dates, nutmeg, clove, gold, pippali (long pepper), shatavari (asparagus root, *Asparagus racemosus*) and licorice root are among the substances used in virilizing recipes. When two people come together to unite themselves sexually they should prepare for themselves a well-appointed bedchamber with Sweet music, Sweet fragrances and Sweet flowers to look at, to nourish and satisfy the mind and all the senses. Flowers are the sex organs of plants, and their presence enhances the effect.

The full moon night is the best of all nights for sexual union, if the woman is not menstruating, because the moon floods the mind with Rasa. Lunar eclipses and new moon nights, on which the natural lunar luminescence is darkened, are meant for meditation, not sexual excitement. Every other night of the month is permissible, and each night the experience will differ, according to the phase of the moon. On whichever night is chosen the couple should don clean, Sweet-smelling clothes after a good bath and should then eat a light meal of Sweet foods with a little wine. Because sex, like exercise, should not be performed immediately after eating, the couple should then engage themselves in dalliance for an hour or more before becoming truly passionate.

All this Sweetness, coupled with a gay, carefree attitude, ensures a wonderful experience and, if conception should occur, a wonderful child. Ancient texts describe at least 84 positions for sexual pleasure. When conception is desired male-on-top positions, which allow the sperm to reach the ovum with least obstruction and make it easier for the zygote to implant itself in the wall of the womb, are best. Whether or not conception is the object of the union the male must maintain firm control of himself so that his partner can satiate herself with pleasure.

After sex you should urinate, to expel any residual Vata from your pelvis, and take a hot bath, to relax your body. It is good to do one or two Yoga asanas to balance Vata. To replenish the Shukra which has been expended both partners should then drink a cup of hot milk cooked with dates and ghee to which slivered almonds, honey and saffron have been added. Milk, ghee and honey all enhance Ojas, but milk is the best of all substances to nourish Shukra quickly. Be sure not to use ghee and honey in equal amounts. If one or both partners are allergic to milk almond milk can be used instead.

Rasayana

Increase in Shukra is also the goal of physical rejuvenation, which requires strict discipline. The effect you obtain is directly proportional to the discipline you follow. Some self-controlled people use discipline alone for rejuvenation, and utilize their inherent Prana, Tejas and Ojas for transmutation. Modern research has proven that there are two guaranteed ways to live longer: decrease your body temperature and decrease your food intake. It has been estimated that a mere 3°F reduction in normal body temperature could make us live an extra 30 years. More years can be added by reducing your food intake to the minimum required for good nutrition. Vitamins and minerals can help, but indirectly. Exercise can strengthen your body and increase its stamina, but not its lifespan.

Some yogis like to sit in meditation for years on end in the intense cold of the High Himalaya, ingesting as little as possible. Their abstemiousness and Yoga and their passive acceptance of the external cold preserves their bodies far more effectively than they would be able to preserve themselves in a polluted, stress-filled environment like a city. Such Yogis differ from us also in the end for which they seek a longer life: to permit them to perfect their meditations.

This is why Yogis worship the great Lord Shiva. Shiva is not a "god" in the normal sense of that English word. He is instead the personification of the power of transformation. Shiva possesses the power to transform anything He likes. He is called the God of Death because His transformations are so intense that most beings who undergo them are unable to maintain their ahamkara-integrity and have no alternative but to dissolve.

Shiva is often portrayed as a Yogi living atop Mt. Kailas, the holiest of all pilgrimage spots for Hindus, Buddhists and Jains alike. Like all peaks in the High Himalaya, Mt. Kailas is intensely cold. Heat causes dilation of all sensory channels, to permit the organism to project its mind into the external world and experience its sense objects. Cold constricts these sensory channels and impedes this projection of mind. When ahamkara is filled with desire for experience she heats up the mind and body to prepare them for sensory experiences. As desire dies mind and body cool, and the senses turn inward.

Ordinary exposure to cold or cold emotions like fear strips fire from an ordinary body, whose heat is diffused throughout all its tissues. Yogis practice Yoga for decades to gradually constrict all their channels evenly and smoothly, concentrating their fire deep within where it is safe from all external influences. They simultaneously refine their internal concentration, aiming to withstand the power of Shiva's transformation. Anyone interested in rejuvenation must learn internal concentration, which my teacher Vimalananda referred to as "interiority."

All mental and physical strain must be eliminated from your life if you hope to rejuvenate yourself through discipline alone. You must cultivate internal and external calm and quiet in a stabilized mind with a firm mental disposition. Some Yogis follow these restrictions alone in their caves in the towering mountains where they are unlikely to be disturbed. If you cannot control your emotions perfectly you will be unable to rejuvenate yourself with discipline alone; fiery emotion will burn away your Ojas as it collects, and frigid emotion will dry it up.

Strict dietary control is an essential part of rejuvenation. You will have to eliminate from your diet the Hot Tastes, which direct the consciousness externally. You will have to avoid alcohol and all other intoxicants, all Pungent, Sour and Salty food and drink, and anger, hatred and all other such divisive emotions. Eliminate Astringency and its accompanying fear to keep your channels of nutrition unconstricted. Even Bitter, which is essential for bringing the doshas into balance, has no place in this diet. Sweet alone is permitted, and the three most important Sweet rejuvenating foods for a discipline-oriented rejuvenation program are fresh cow's milk, cow's ghee and honey.

Perfect physical and mental discipline is one way of withdrawing from the world. When you simply refuse to allow provocation to affect you, you might as well be living in a cave in the Himalaya. If you find yourself still falling prey to occasional emotional upset you will need to physically retreat from the world for some time, to learn how not to react to provocations that might otherwise agitate your mind and burn your Ojas. If you cannot retreat from the world forever you should arrange to retreat for at least a month, during which time you should use a rejuvenating substance to enhance the effect of your discipline. V and P types usually need substances, Vs because their dryness exhausts Ojas and Ps because their inner fire burns Ojas. One month is really a minimum to obtain any kind of significant effect, although any retreat of any length, even a day, is bound to be beneficial.

Ideally, you should avoid all human contact during your retreat, remaining in your room, avoiding even wind and sun. Isolation from the external world helps you balance your internal existence. Thorough panchakarma purification is needed before you begin your retreat, and careful regulation of your food and sleep is essential during it. Sex is banned during the rejuvenation period. This may sound boring, but rejuvenation cannot occur in an atmosphere of perpetual stimulation and excitement. You cannot be "busy" rejuvenating any more than a tree can be busy growing. Rejuvenation, like growth, happens at Nature's pace.

A rejuvenating substance can enhance the effects of your discipline even if you are unable to go on retreat. You should consume it early in the morning, well before breakfast, so it need not compete with food for digestion. You must consume the substance for at least three weeks for it to have any effect; six weeks is better. During this period you must avoid everything you would avoid during convalescence, including extensive travel, loud or extensive speaking, violent behavior and any other Vata-disturbing activities that would destroy Ojas. Meditation and mild exercise are desirable.

Some simple rejuvenating formulas:

Crush seven *black peppercorns* and mix their powder with honey. Yogis like black pepper because its drying effect dries reproductive secretions and helps preserve celibacy. It also dries other body secretions, and is a good rejuvenator for those who have weak lungs that are easily clogged by Kapha. Black pepper is better for K, VK and PK types than it is for Vs, VPs and Ps.

Pippali (long pepper) is a specific rejuvenator for the lungs. Though Pungent in Taste and Hot in Energy it is Sweet in Post-Digestive Effect. Because it is oily it can increase Kapha if used continuously for several months. Misuse of pippali can increase all Three Doshas.

Soak one handful of *chickpeas* overnight in water. Next morning slowly chew and swallow them after rinsing off their skins. Some people wash them down with the soak water. This practice is especially good for weakness of the stomach.

Gently heat 1 tsp. of *powdered licorice root* in one cup of milk; do not boil. Drink twice daily. If you have high blood pressure avoid long-term use of licorice root, which can cause the body to retain water. Licorice root is especially good for the sexual organs.

Shatavari, a variety of asparagus root, is especially rejuvenative for the female reproductive organs. One tsp. simmered 5 to 10 minutes in a cup of milk with 1/4 tsp. powdered ginger and a finely chopped date is good for both V and P types.

Ashvagandha (Withania somnifera), which is sometimes called the "Indian ginseng," is particularly rejuvenating for men. It is also aphrodisiac and forms a good addition to the shatavari milk recipe above.

Garlic is especially rejuvenating for V and K types. It has five Tastes—all except Sour—but Pungent and Sweet predominate. It is Hot in Energy and Pungent in Post-Digestive Effect. Green garlic, which is plucked after only a couple of weeks of life when it has its first long green leaves and is used as the whole plant, is much milder, far less likely to aggravate Pitta, and much less disturbing to the mind than is ordinary garlic. Always reduce dry garlic's intensity by sautéing it for 30 seconds in ghee or unsalted butter before using it. P and V types can also simmer it 5 to 10 minutes in a cup milk mixed with 1/2 cup water, then strain and drink.

Tulsi, or holy basil (*Ocimum sanctum*), is said to possess an unusually strong form of prana within it that can treat almost any disease, including some forms of cancer. It is ideal for fevers. For prevention of dosha imbalance V and K types can take one ounce of the juice of the fresh leaves each morning.

Pomegranate juice is rejuvenating on its own, or it can be carefully evaporated into a thick syrup over a low fire. Daily one silver leaf and one gold leaf can be added to two tsp. of this syrup and the mixture made into a ball. This ball is then consumed with fresh milk.

Gotu kola (Hydrocotyle asiatica), known in India as *brahmi,* helps rejuvenate the mind and improve the memory. It is mainly Bitter in Taste, with Astringent and Sweet aftertastes, Cold Energy and Sweet Post-Digestive Effect. Overuse of gotu kola can occasionally increase Vata. Gotu kola is best for V types and P types if its tea is simmered gently with ghee until all the water disappears so that its active principles remain in the ghee. This prevents any side-effects. K types should take it as a tea.

Triphala paste can be applied to the bottom of a clean new cast iron pan to permit it to absorb some of the iron. After at least 24 hours it can be removed, one tsp. at a time, and consumed as a paste with honey followed by a glass of warm water in which one tsp. of honey has been dissolved. This is especially good for those who need to eliminate large quantities of ama which have accumulated over many years.

Haritaki is sometimes used alone or in preparations like *Agastya Rasayana* to scrape away ama and rejuvenate simultaneously. Haritaki can cause Vata increase if used continuously for too long. It should not be given to emaciated, dried-out individuals, pregnant women, or to people who have a Pitta imbalance or who have recently hemorrhaged. It should be given with raw sugar during summer or in a hot climate, and with dry ginger or long pepper during winter or in a cold climate. In autumn, it should be mixed with rock salt, and in spring with honey.

Amalaki fruit when fresh is most often made into jam or preserves. *Amalaki Rasayana* and *Dhatri Rasayana* are two common preparations. The most famous of all amalaki-based rejuvenators is *Chyavana Prasha Avaleha*. Amalaki is its main ingredient, supported by more than two dozen other herbs added for synergistic effects. A sweetener, such as raw sugar, jaggery (solidified sugar cane juice) or honey is added to provide intense, concentrated Sweet. Amalaki and the other herbs insure that the Sweet is properly digested and causes no reaction.

The dose of Chyavana Prasha is 1 to 2 Tbsp. each morning, followed by a cup of warm milk with saffron. Always add saffron after removing the milk from the fire, to preserve its potency. A good way to consume Chyavana Prasha is with the help of dried dates, which you can obtain from an Indian grocery store. Soak two of these dates overnight. Next morning slit open the swollen dates and fill them with Chyavana Prasha and a blanched almond. Chew slowly.

Minerals and Metals

Minerals have been probably been used in Ayurveda since its beginning, but their prominence expanded dramatically when Tantra began its researches into alchemy. Every mineral, like every herb, has its own Taste-personality. Gold, for example, is Sweet, silver is Sour, copper Pungent, and iron Astringent. Gold is an ideal medicine for Vata because it is Hot as well as Sweet. Silver is a good remedy for Pitta because like amalaki it is Cold as well as Sour; while its Sourness increases the digestive fire, its Cold prevents Pitta from increasing. Copper controls Kapha, being both Hot and Pungent, and scrapes ama and Kapha from the body. Iron, which nourishes Blood, prevents Blood from becoming too Hot or too fluid with its Astringency.

Gold is spoken of alchemically as solidified sunrays, for its effects on living organisms are like those of the sun. Wearing gold purifies all energy entering the body, improves the skin and the body's overall beauty, and strengthens the joints and the being's overall energy. Gold is a general antidote for all types of poison, including ama. Gold also controls Vata and helps eliminate ama from the system. The gold salts used in modern medicine to treat arthritis cause side-effects because they are soluble. They dissolve into reactive ions that are too intense to be safely utilized by the system.

Ayurvedic metals and minerals, including gold, are prepared in a very different way. First they are thoroughly purified, to remove any poisonous pollutants. Then pastes of medicinal herbs are applied to them and they are incinerated. Some scientists believe that the herbs form chelates with the minerals; others have different theories. What is certain is that after the incineration most of these minerals, except gold and probably silver, become oxides or sulfides.

Most metal oxides and sulfides are quite insoluble in water and so do not break up into reactive ions when they enter the body. Though they remain chemically unreactive within the body they seem to exert a catalytic effect on metabolic processes. Gold, and silver to a great extent, apparently remain unreacted, but the incineration reduces them into particles of colloidial size or smaller which remain chemically inert. Other metals are converted into oxides or sulfides to eliminate their reactivity; gold, which is practically non-reactive anyway, needs only to be finely divided.

More incinerations means smaller particle size. When the particles become sufficiently small, at least small enough to fill the lines on the fingertips, they can circulate in the system and exert their effects much longer than can ordinary medicines. This is one of the reasons that minerals are useful for rejuvenation therapy. Another reason: *Bhasmas* (incinerated metals and minerals) become more potent with age as their particles naturally become smaller and smaller, whereas herbs lose their potency after a year or two. 100-year-old bhasmas are highly prized in India.

The dose of a bhasma is commonly a small heap of powder the size of a grain of rice. The Taste of the bhasma is intense, but usually less unpleasant than that of some of Ayurveda's intensely bitter herbal products. Bhasmas also act more quickly than herbs, and their effects tend to last longer. For quick results a bhasma is made into a paste with honey, butter or ghee and the paste is then placed under the tongue. A bhasma's first effect comes from the transmission of its Taste into the brain; its second effect, which it delivers almost as quickly as its first, involves the release of Prana into the bloodstream, carried by a subtle, potentiated form of oxygen created during the process of incineration. The third effect, the one due to the mineral itself, occurs as the particles of the bhasma circulate throughout the body.

Each physician traditionally prepared his or her own medicines, but with cultural modernization many physicians have elected to rely on Ayurvedic pharmaceutical manufacturers to provide them with medicaments. As Ayurvedic medicines become more available outside India the question of their quality will become more and more acute. "Know your dealer" is an important watchword even today for those who would purchase Ayurvedic medicines in India. Many Ayurvedic pharmacies produce bhasmas nowadays; not all of them produce them well.

For example, mica (*abhraka* in Sanskrit) bhasma is an excellent rejuvenator for the lungs and for Rasa Dhatu. To make the best mica bhasma you must dig a hole in the ground three feet cubical and lay aside a store of 1500 cakes of dried cow dung. Cow dung cakes are used widely in India as fuel and to cremate corpses because they burn slowly with intense heat. After filling the pit with about 500 cakes you add a sealed clay vessel containing the mica and its herbal helpers, then finish filling the pit with the other 1000 cakes. It will take at least a day for the pile to burn itself out. After it cools you retrieve and open the clay vessel, extract the mica, and prepared it with fresh herbs for its next incineration. All told it takes two or three days to perform one incineration properly and prepare for the next.

Like most minerals, mica requires only 5, 7, or 11 incinerations to make it minimally fit for use. But "minimally fit" is a long way from "superb." Mica bhasma becomes powerful after 100 incinerations, and superbly puissant after 1000 firings. Yogis who had unlimited time, herbs and cow dung could afford to invest the half-dozen or more years it takes to properly incinerate mica 1000 times. Modern companies cannot afford to do so, so they simplify the process and use electric furnaces to do the job more quickly. Mica bhasma prepared this way becomes minimally fit sooner than that prepared the traditional fashion, but does not improve exponentially with each subsequent firing as its cow-dung-fired counterpart. Those who use commercially-prepared mica bhasma may as well use that which has been incinerated just enough to lose all its sparkle, in a larger dose than otherwise would be necessary.

Likewise, many companies tout their diamond bhasma as a panacea for all ills including cancer. Not too many people know how to make diamond bhasma properly, however. Unless you are an expert you are as likely to be cheated over diamond bhasma as you are over gem-quality diamonds. For this reason substitutes have been identified. If you are unable to obtain reliable diamond bhasma you can use bhasma of other gemstones such as tourmaline instead, and reap almost the same benefit. If gold bhasma is beyond the reach of your pocketbook you can use bhasma of pyrites (suvarna makshika, mentioned in the discussion on arthritis) instead because it is also a rejuvenator for Rasa Dhatu.

Even properly prepared bhasmas can be dangerous if they are overused, and if improperly used they may have no effect. Vimalananda was once called upon to consult with a Maharaja. This ruler's court physicians, all well-trained Ayurvedic doctors, had been treating him for weeks with a bhasma without any result. Vimalananda examined the prescription and found it to be correct, and then asked about diet. When he found that the Maharaja was still eating salt

Vimalananda told him to stop it, and in a matter of days the disease disappeared.

Some minerals are not incinerated. Shilajit, a black tarlike substance that exudes from mountains in hot weather, is an ingredient in rejuvenating compounds such as Chandra Prabha, which is useful in many conditions including diabetes, obesity and urinary tract complaints. Shilajit strengthens the immune system, regulates the menstrual cycle, and tones the male reproductive organs. Shilajit is also used dissolved with other herbs and honey in hot milk to promote physical and mental strength and virility.

Since bhasmas are still generally unavailable some metals can be used in their pure forms. Bracelets of pure copper, for example, are indeed good for rheumatism, as folk wisdom in this country has had it for years, because the copper scrapes ama away from the tissues. Only V and K people can use such bracelets, however; copper is too hot for Ps. Copper or even gold may burn a P person's skin when worn. If copper leaves a green discoloration on your skin it indicates that your system is already quite hot and acidic and needs no copper.

If you cannot wear your desired metal you can drink your water from a copper or a silver glass, or boil a piece of 24-carat gold in water for about half an hour and then take the resulting water in doses of 1 tsp. You can also put a piece of a purified metal on your photograph, or on a lock of your cut hair, to provide you with vibrations from the metal without introducing it physically into your body.

Some modern scientists claim that calamus root (*Acorus calamus*) is carcinogenic. Many Indians, however, insert a thin wire of 24-carat gold into a longitudinal hole in a whole calamus root and then rub the root clockwise into 1/2 tsp. of honey on a flat surface. 3 rubs is the dose for a child, and 7 or more for an adult. This paste is given to a child from birth until 3 to 6 months of age to activate the immune system, which gold does better than anything else because it is so Sweet and so nourishing to all the dhatus.

Makaradhwaja

Vimalananda taught me about the power of gold by reminding me that it is mined with the help of cyanide. Anything that can dissolve gold must have a deep affinity for the yellow metal. Gold is a highly concentrated Sweet, a powerful nutrient for body, mind and aura. It is tonic and rejuvenating, and it is possible that the tonic and rejuvenating effects of such substances as yarrow, bamboo, almonds and apricots may be due to the tiny amounts of cyanogens (substances which release cyanide) which they contain.

Larger doses of cyanide kill by interfering with cellular respiration, the release of energy caused by the combination of oxygen with various substances inside a cell. Cells die when their energy sources are cut off. Gold (and presumably small doses of cyanide) exerts the opposite effect of making cellular respiration more efficient so that it yields more energy with less waste.

Everyone's aura tells a different story of immune preparedness, but golden is the healthiest color for an aura. The most common Sanskrit word for gold, *suvarna,* literally means "beautiful color." Intake of the solidified sunrays that make up gold will surely gild your aura, provided of course that you can digest those rays.

Gold by itself may be difficult to digest, especially if it so inflames your physical fire of digestion that you begin to ignore your physical limits and overindulge yourself. It is best to consume gold only after it has been first digested—by the metal mercury. Gold is mercury's food, and when gold is administered with mercury the likelihood of its being properly digested by the body improves dramatically.

Mercury is described as the semen of Lord Shiva, which means that mercury is the embodiment on the physical plane of the fire of transformation. Mercury can provide tremendous Tejas to any organism, and can make that organism digest almost anything. Since mercury is semen, or Shukra, it is the ultimate aphrodisiac, the supreme virilizer. Semen is alive, full of Prana, and mercury can similarly provide Prana to the system. Shukra being the raw material from which Ojas is produced, mercury can create unlimited Ojas in an organism. Mercury thus provides the body with all three essentials for life—Prana, Tejas, and Ojas—and thus possesses the potential to control all Three Doshas.

Mercury, which is of course a deadly poison, must be carefully purified before it is used in medicine. Even after purification mercury is too powerful to use in metallic form, however. Most commonly it is reacted with sulfur to form black sulfide of mercury, which after heating becomes red sulfide of mercury. Sulfur is the menstrual blood of Shiva's wife Parvati, the only substance that can properly control mercury's tremendous power. Since sulfur is a form of Blood which can create other beings, it is as if sulfur acts as the womb in which the mercurial semen develops into the new child: Kajjali, black sulfide of mercury.

Sulfur's affinity for heavy metals has long been known. The active portion of BAL, the first drug developed to remove heavy metals from the body, is two sulfur atoms. Black sulfide of mercury is almost totally insoluble in either water or weak acids, and so the potential for poisoning by free mercury is very low. Red sulfide of mercury is slightly more soluble, but its potential for causing toxicity is also low. In fact, mercury sulfide's innate safety is recognized even today, for it is used industrially to help scavenge stray elemental mercury.

There is no disease which mercury cannot cure if it is properly prepared and used, say the texts, and if it is improperly prepared or misused there is no disease it cannot cause. No proof of the second half of the ancient saying is necessary; all of us know how poisonous mercury is. The first half of the saying has been proved over centuries of safe use of mercury in Ayurvedic medicines. When side-effects arise from mercurial medications they may result from impurities which were not removed before the mercury is processed or from improper processing. Anyone who wants to use mercury for rejuvenation must be exceptionally careful about its source, and must be sure that it has been properly prepared. No one should **ever** even **think** of trying to prepare mercury for internal use without proper training!

The quantity of mercury in any one Ayurvedic pill is very small, thanks to the processing procedure known as bhavana. In bhavana an herbal decoction or juice is added to a small amount of the medicinal substance and the resulting mixture is rubbed slowly in a mortar and pestle until it dries. The smooth, gentle, continuous motion provides a smooth, gentle vibration to the medicine, and the rubbing and grinding reduce its particle size, thus improving its effectiveness. Each bhavana reduces the mercurial concentration of the finished product and potentizes it, in much the same way as homeopathic medicines are potentized.

The most renowned of all mercurial rejuvenators is Makaradhwaja, whose main ingredients are mercury, sulfur and gold. Makaradhwaja regenerates vigor and vitality, improves immunity, and assists in body development by increasing metabolic activity. Makaradhwaja benefits all sorts of acute disease states, including especially respiratory ailments like cold, influenza, pneumonia and asthma, and all sorts of general conditions such as low blood pressure, general exhaustion and nervous or mental debility. It can keep the whole being alert and energetic well into old age.

The best forms of Makaradhwaja have gold leaf on the outer surface of the pill as well as gold within. The dose of Makaradhwaja is usually one pill once or twice a day, crushed and made into a paste with honey or Chyavana Prasha, and washed down with a cup of warm milk and saffron. This should be taken at least 1/2 hour before meals, and should be continued for 3 to 6 weeks. It is usually best to take Makaradhwaja and other mercury-based rejuvenators during the coldest season of the year so that their powerful innate fire does not increase Pitta. Two cycles of mercury-based medicine each year are sufficient for most people.

Other Rasayanas

Other mercury-based rejuvenators include:

Parpati - black sulfide of mercury prepared into a thick film. Parpati tones and enlivens the membrane lining the colon, improving its ability to absorb Prana from ingested food. Gold, mica, iron, copper and herbs are added to some Parpati compounds to achieve specific therapeutic effects.

Lakshmi Vilasa Rasa - its main ingredients, beyond mercury sulfide, are gold, silver, mica, copper, tin, iron, pearls and aconite. Its rejuvenating effect concentrates on the heart and lungs and the dhatus Rasa and Blood. It is particularly good for bronchial asthma.

Vasanta Kusumakara Rasa - its main ingredients are almost the same as in Lakshmi Vilasa Rasa, but its effects differ because of different bhavanas. Vasanta Kusumakara undergoes 35 or more bhavanas of such varied substances as cow's milk, sugar cane juice, jasmine flower juice, sandalwood tea and musk water. It improves the body's ability to digest Rasa, which makes it effective therapeutically in diabetes, heart disease and consumption. It is a strong virilizer.

Suvarna Malini Vasanta – is one of a class of three closely related compounds (the other two being Laghu Malini Vasanta and Madhu Malini Vasanta) which act mainly on consumption. Suvarna Malini Vasanta contains gold, pearls, mercury sulfide, white pepper and a form of zinc called *kharpara*, which like both black and white pepper dries excessive secretions, especially in the respiratory tract. 21 bhavanas of lime juice are performed to these ingredients, followed by one bhavana of fresh butter to prevent the result from being too drying.

Their drying effects make these three compounds useful in all sorts of diseases of Rasa Dhatu including chronic bronchitis, pleurisy, fever, consumption, leucorrhea and anemia. It enhances the vision, helps build strong fetuses, and promotes the expulsion of ama and other poisons from the system. In spite of its drying effect it can reverse the weight and energy loss which might occur after a serious disease or in old age.

Suvarna Raja Vangeshvara - although its color is metallic golden it contains no gold. Its main constituents are mercury, sulfur and tin. Ammonium chloride is used as a flux, and the mixture is heated in a glass vial on a sand bath. In this instance the desired result drops to the bottom of the vial, suggesting a strong action on the lower parts of the body, which is indeed the case. Suvarna Raja Vangeshvara is most effective in loss of Shukra, as from frequent masturbation or wet dreams, and in conditions like consumption when they result from loss of Shukra. Impotence and premature ejaculation also respond, as do certain forms of diabetes.

Smrti Sagara Rasa - this pill, whose name means "Ocean of Memory," is one of several Ayurvedic preparations that contain arsenic compounds. Arsenic, which is essential to human nutrition in small amounts, is found naturally in such foods as almonds, barley, carrots, corn, grapes, oats, pineapples and rice. It is used in Indian medicine mainly as a powerful invigorator. Arsenic's oxide, being quite poisonous, is less commonly used than are its sulfides. Smrti Sagara Rasa contains mercury sulfide, copper oxide, arsenic bisulfide and arsenic trisulfide in just sufficient quantities to gently stimulate the memory. This mixture is then processed with some well-known brain tonics: 21 bhavanas each of calamus root tea and gotu kola juice, and one bhavana of jyotishmati oil.

Hema Garbha - containing mercury sulfide, gold, and copper oxide, this medicine is simmered in liquefied sulfur in an earthenware crucible and made into a stick which is rubbed into a paste with honey on a stone. Hema Garbha is a powerful rejuvenator and heart tonic which is given sublingually in extreme Vata disturbances like coma.

These are only a few of the many Ayurvedic rejuvenators available. It is impossible to overstate the dangers inherent in self-dosing yourself with any of these substances. Never experiment with any of them on your own; consume them only under the direct supervision of a qualified Ayurvedic physician.

Seasons

A Sufi from Bombay once gave me his prescription for good health. "Most of the time," he said, "I live a strict life, and always eat at home. But once a month I make it a point to go to a restaurant and eat a good meal. Eating regularly in restaurants is not healthy, I know, but at least once a month it is good to do so. This way I expose my system to all the diseases that are prevalent in the community. Then my immune system is prepared for anything that might otherwise sneak up on me unawares."

This is good advice. It is unwise to try to live too pure a life nowadays. There are just too many pollutants around us, in our air, water and food, for us to be totally pristine. Even if you should happen to succeed at thoroughly purifying yourself today, your environment will begin to pollute you again tomorrow. Purification cannot be done once and then forgotten about. Ayurveda mandates regular purification for preventative maintenance, followed by rejuvenation to counteract the recurrent destabilizations of life.

Try as we may to insulate ourselves from the influence of external forces with humidifiers, air conditioners and central heaters, we expose ourselves to our environments every time we leave our cocoons. This continual reorientation causes continual stress. In attempting to create a standard year-round environment we have engineered instead a year-round source of physical aggravation and imbalance.

All constitutional weaknesses are strongly influenced by time. Vata-caused problems, for example, always worsen "when clouds fill the sky," much as our old timers claim that the appearance of aches and pains in their rheumatic joints forecasts a storm. Any change of weather is likely to disturb Vata, since Vata is aggravated by change, but each constitution is affected differently during each season. "Season" includes all sorts of time cycles:

Vata predominates: after digestion, during assimilation
during the pre-dawn and late afternoon hours
during autumn and early winter in old age

Pitta predominates:	during digestion
	at midday and midnight
	during summer
	in middle age
Kapha predominates:	after eating before digestion begins
	at daybreak and nightfall
	during late winter and spring
	in childhood and youth

A V person will naturally find it more difficult to maintain balance when Vata predominates in a season since the environment itself will reinforce Vata's ·strength. P people similarly will tend to find Pitta increasing within them dramatically during Pitta-predominant periods, and even K people may find Kapha seasons hard to negotiate. Autumn is often the worst season for Vs because the weather is most changeable then, and because wind storms like hurricanes and tornados are prevalent. V people should avoid beginning major new projects in the fall, and even if they bend their dietary and lifestyle rules during the rest of the year they should renew their harmony-producing discipline in autumn. Ps must be strictest with themselves during summer or whenever else it is exceedingly hot. K people most need discipline in spring, when the snow melts and the sap runs in Nature, and the Kapha flows in the body.

Everyone must be alert, however, to prevent imbalance during the "joints" between these seasons, the periods when one season is changing into another and the "weather" is not sure itself which season it belongs to. This external confusion in Nature is mirrored by internal confusion in the organism. Spring fever, for example, can strike anyone, and is due to the inertia carried by the powerful flow of Kapha that happens at the end of winter.

Regular purification can control this. Since Kapha predominates in the spring, removing excess Kapha when winter has died but spring has not yet quite been born can prevent diseases due to Kapha accumulation. Excess Pitta should be eliminated in the interim between spring and summer, and excess Vata between summer and fall.

India's Rishis created festivals and traditions to encourage everyone to remember to change their diets and habits as the seasons changed. For example, one of India's several New Year's Days falls each year on the day after the New Moon that is nearest to the vernal equinox. It is traditional in Western India to rise early on that day and eat a few neem leaves before consuming anything else. The myth says that doing this will prevent any bitterness in your life during the rest of the year. One message hidden in this myth is that there need be no Bitterness due to disease if neem (or a similarly Bitter substance) is used during that season to control Kapha (which is predominant then) and to discourage Pitta from accumulating (since Pitta becomes predominant as the weather warms up).

According to Indian astrology, the sun moves into the constellation of Capricorn on January 14. All over Western India people wander around on this day handing one another confections made of sesame seeds and jaggery (solidified sugar cane juice), saying "Eat sesame jaggery so that you will speak sweetly!" Sesame seeds, especially the black variety, are nourishing and virilizing but difficult to digest. Since the body's digestive fire is strongest in the winter, when extra food is needed to keep warm, consumption of black sesame seeds and jaggery then helps preserve the body's strength. When you add this (or a similar supplement) to your diet during the cold season your sense organs will become better able to function ("speak") efficiently ("sweetly") during the coming months of aggravated doshas. Time is an important factor in the life of every mortal, and living according to Nature's time is the only way to remain healthy.

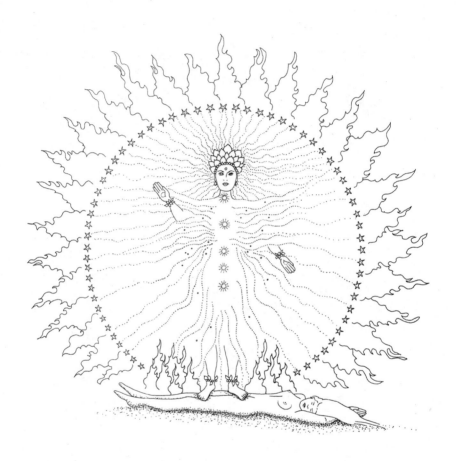

BEYOND AYURVEDA

Chapter Nine
Beyond Ayurveda

Immortality

Ahamkara uses body and mind for her gratification as long as she can, but even with good rejuvenation every organism eventually wears out. Dependence on the external universe for any kind of nourishment—physical, mental, emotional or spiritual—causes wear and tear. Mind, senses and spirit cannot be satisfied by "bread alone"; they must feel *prasanna*, "satisfied," to be healthy. As long as they believe themselves to need sensory gratification to be satisfied they will maintain their external orientation, searching the outside world for gratification.

Mind and spirit need not be wholly dependent on the body. One study of 600 individuals with hydrocephalus, a condition in which 95% of the volume of the skull is filled with cerebro-spinal fluid instead of brain tissue, found 300 of them to have IQs greater than 100, indicating above average intelligence. If the mind can function without most of its brain it should also be able to function without many of the other things we think it requires. The rishis understood this, and because they wanted to go beyond the limitations of time they realized that reliance on external sustenance makes an individual subject to time.

They also knew that each season has its own Taste, which permeates the food, water and air available to us during that season. Since Taste influences emotion, and since mortals are dependent on external sources of juice, they realized that their mental balance was also dependent on the influences of the seasonal changes of the environment.

They therefore restricted themselves first to roots and fruits, then to milk, then to water, and finally solely to air, to eliminate the negative physical and mental effects that all physical food possesses. They learned how to obtain their Prana from the air, and how to create all dhatus and ultimately even Ojas directly from this Prana with the help of the powerful Tejas enkindled in them by their spiritual austerities. This permitted them to escape from the influence of external juice, and made them immortal.

An immortal does not need to eat physical food. His or her organism can create all Six Tastes internally, within itself, in the proper proportions needed for ahamkara's self-expression. Immortality is true freedom, freedom from all limitations. A mortal cannot simply decide one day to do without food altogether; the system has to adapt itself very slowly to a food-free existence.

The food we eat provides us a very crude form of Prana. That Prana which comes in with each breath through the nostrils is much finer, but is still crude compared to that which can be obtained through the eyes by such processes as *trataka*, concentrated staring at flames or the sun. The supreme form of Prana is that which is imbibed by the mind directly from the universe telepathically, without the interposition of any sense organ. These subtler forms of Prana are much Sweeter than Prana from normal sources. They require little digestion, satiate body and mind more profoundly, and can be imbibed only through internal concentration. Thus the Yogis speak of enjoying *jnanamrtam bhojanam*, "the sustenance of the nectar of knowledge."

Even those of us who lack the perfect internal concentration to obtain these finer forms of Prana can obtain refined Prana from mercury. One interpretation of the word rasayana is "the Path of Mercury." Rasashastra, the "Science of Rasa," is the art of purifying and controlling mercury to utilize its power to evaporate the effects of aging. Since crude mercury is far too poisonous to accomplish this task, Prana is first added to mercury that has been preliminarily purified. Then that mercury is brought to life, awakened, instructed, fed, bound, swooned and sacrificed. These refining processes are called *samskaras.*

The word samskara is closely related to the word Sanskrit, which is actually spelled *Samskrta*, "that which has undergone samskara." Sanskrit is not an ordinary language, one that evolved by trial and error over centuries of mass mispronunciation. Sanskrit is a product of phonetic engineering. Each of its words has a vibratory meaning in addition to its overt meaning. This is why Sanskrit is called a *mantric* language, a language whose each word is a mantra. A *mantra* is a group of sounds which when pronounced in a particular way creates a particular vibration in the brain and body of the pronouncer and on anything into which the pronouncer directs it.

Just as food can carry prayer or hatred into the system, a mantra's vibration can be carried on any substance, even water, into the body. Because mantras are much subtler than physical fire and grinding, medicines that have been prepared with mantras exert a profounder effect on the whole organism than any ordinary medicines can. Samskaras on mercury were originally performed with both herbs and mantras, and the medicines thus produced were exponentially more powerful than are today's commercially prepared medicines whose samskaras are performed with herbs alone.

One Sanskrit word for mercury is *parada*, that which carries you to the far shore of existence and makes you immortal. It is also called *rasa*, because it has a perfect complement of Six Tastes. Yogis say that while herbs can keep you alive for 400 to 500 years, mercury can keep you alive forever, if you understand the discipline and restrictions behind its use. Mercury is the sole metal or mineral that can actually be brought to life. The alchemist creates life in mercury and then takes it again; he sacrifices the mercury to obtain its Prana.

Sacrifice

External alchemy, which developed from the internal alchemy of Tantra, is like all else in the Vedic universe rooted in the concept of sacrifice. At the beginning of time the Cosmic Being's ahamkara surrendered His own body to be dismembered, and each portion of those remains developed into one aspect of the cosmos. To become immortal is to become the Supreme Being of your internal universe, and anyone who succeeds at becoming immortal must emulate the sacrifice of that original Cosmic Being. Immortals sacrifice themselves spontaneously when their gratitude to Nature at permitting them to become deathless so overflows them that they realize that they have nothing left to hold onto. They open their final barriers of self to Nature, who then enters them and begins to direct their every move. Immortals offer all action as a sacrifice to nourish Nature and to remedy the imbalances that Her other children cause in Her. Immortals sacrifice themselves ceaselessly to promote and preserve the health of the body politic.

Ahamkara is addicted to food. Most of us are addicted to physical food; saints and sages eliminate ordinary addictions and addict themselves to God. Addiction is the basis for all disorder and disharmony, and addiction to God is the only permanent cure. Addiction to God eliminates all possibility of interference from other beings, because body, mind and spirit all concentrate on the same object. This makes you disease-free, for disease can only arise in the presence of some alien influence. When all becomes God, what remains alien? Even if you are not yet immortal, you can transform your existence if you will but transfer your addictions to God.

Shiva, Vishnu and all the other Indian deities are cosmic forces. The rishis assigned them personalities based on the emotions they create within us. A deity's emotion-personality is just like the Taste-personality that a food or a medicine displays. If you know how to adapt a personality to your condition you can make use of its tastes or emotions to balance your system. Herbs and minerals are also cosmic forces, but they are limited by being physical. A deity's personality comes much closer to being unlimited. Meditation on a cosmic personality concentrates and directs its force into you, transforming your own personality until it comes to resemble your object of concentration.

For example, Krishna, who is an aspect of Vishnu, is Sweetness personified. Everything Krishna touches becomes Sweet (*madhura*) because Krishna Himself is *Madhu*, the unlimited, unqualified cosmic Sweetness. Everyone who makes proper use of Krishna's mantra, even those who do not believe in deities and who doubt Krishna's history, can drink from the bottomless well of permanently satisfying Sweetness which Krishna personifies.

The Vedic, Puranic and Tantric spiritual disciplines, which are inaccurately referred to collectively as the Hindu religion, present a combined physical and mental approach to enhanced spiritual development. Guggulu, Ayurveda's premier anti-inflammatory and cholesterol reducer, has been burned as an incense since Vedic times because of its ability to chase away "evil influences" from a dwelling. While offering Guggulu sacrificially acts on ethereal parasites it has also been shown to kill germs in the air of a room fumigated with its smoke.

Specific herbs have been associated with specific deities for millennia: wood apple (*bilva*, or *Aegle marmelos*) with Shiva and Lakshmi, coconut with Lakshmi, holy basil (*tulasi*) with Vishnu, Bermuda grass with Ganesha, and so on. These herbs give physical, mental and spiritual benefits to devotees who use them properly. For example, Bermuda grass controls blood sugar. Elephants, who love to eat Sweet food, also love Bermuda grass. Bermuda grass keeps elephants from going out of balance when they consume too much Sweet, and can do similar things for the humans who use it. While even crude Bermuda grass is medically beneficial, its medical effect is multiplied manyfold when it is first sacrificed to Ganesha before being used.

Or consider the ritual worship known as the *Satya Narayana Puja*, in which 1000 leaves of tulasi are ritually offered with appropriate mantas to Vishnu. Vishnu is the Preserver, the cosmic force that perpetuates life, and Tulasi in embodied form is said to be one of Vishnu's wives. Tulasi the plant is thus one of the vehicles of the universe's Vishnu power, which suggests that tulasi is one of the best of all substances for preserving life.

Most people today in India perform the Satya Narayana Puja mechanically, unaware of its hidden significance. When at ritual's end the tulasi leaves are collected, the person who organized the worship consumes a handful of them and then digs into the other offering, a big bowl of shira (a sweet porridge made of wheat groats cooked in ghee). If they eat too much shira, which is not unusual after having to sit through a long ritual session, it will either put them to sleep or give them a stomachache.

People who are in the know, however, know that the Satya Narayana Puja is a process of potentizing tulasi leaves to increase their life-extending effects so they can act as a rejuvenator for the individual who consumes them. This potentiation is comparable to the potentiation provided by bhavana and incineration, but mantras are used solely instead of any specialized physical processing. Knowledgeable people will extract (with mantras) the juice from all one thousand consecrated leaves and will consume it (with mantras) along with a small dish of shira. Then the consecrated tulasi juice and shira can work together to provide a rejuvenating effect, the tulasi enkindling the physical and mental digestive fires and the shira providing just the right amount of nourishment for these fires to digest.

The rishis who wrote the Satya Narayana Puja were spiritual researchers. They intuited both tulasi's qualities and the appropriate sounds that could enhance these qualities, and combined them together into a recipe for physical, mental and spiritual development. Potentiation by mantra is as scientific as any other form of potentiation, though it is much subtler. Even if you are a Christian or a Muslim, or you oppose paganism for some other reason, you can still use the Satya Narayana Puja to improve your physical health. Faith in the ritual's esoteric significance enhances its effects, but some effect will be produced no matter what you think of it, if the mantras are pronounced correctly. Mantras are impersonal bundles of power, which become more comprehensible to us when we make use of the transcendent personalities that the rishis have provided to accompany them.

Kundalini

You can use mercury as a rejuvenator even if you cannot bring yourself to believe that it is Lord Shiva's semen. To walk the path of mercury and get the most you can out of it, however, there is no substitute for the worship of Shiva. Lord Shiva dwells in every human being, deep in the brain, in the form of pure, unalloyed consciousness. True immortality is possible only when your personal Shiva has complete control over His *Shakti* (power), which is your ahamkara. So long as this shakti remains in ordinary time-bound mundane consciousness, identifying herself continually with your body and your limited personality, we call her ahamkara, and she creates I-ness for you. Human life exists only because ahamkara deludes herself into believing that she and the limited body-mind personality are identical.

Once ahamkara starts to awaken from her slumber of ignorance, however, she realizes that she is not the same as the limited, impermanent you. She can no longer pretend that you are everything to her. At this stage we begin to call her by a different name: Kundalini. As Kundalini awakens she realizes that she is Shiva's Shakti, and will try to rush back up the spine to reunite with Him. Should she awaken completely in someone who has not already undergone strenuous penance that person will be transported beyond normal mundane time into infinity by this experience. In such circumstances the body cannot continue to exist; Kundalini will forget it entirely, and will remember only Shiva. The moment that she sacrifices her identity to Him she undergoes instant enlightenment.

If instead like a good Yogi you have used the Shiva-consciousness to prepare your physical, mental and spiritual being for this tremendous evolutionary experience there is a chance that you will be able to retain your body, at least for a time. If you have become immortal you can keep your body forever, and can instruct your Kundalini to identify with it or with Shiva at your whim. This is absolute health, total control of ahamkara and its immune defenses.

Many people follow spiritual disciplines, hoping to become enlightened through meditation and other austerities. Most of these people do so with only a hazy knowledge of physical and mental physiology; very few of them know anything at all about Ayurveda. Sometimes they experiment with powers like Kundalini of which they know little. Being the source of embodied life itself Kundalini is the most powerful of all medicines. She can cure all ailments when properly approached, and can cause all ailments when improperly employed.

If you are physically and mentally unprepared for this forcible ripping away of ahamkara from its safe haven in your limited human body and attendant personality you may suffer severe, permanent physical and psychic damage as a result of Kundalini's partial awakening. The "Kundalini crisis," a disease in which Kundalini's power is unleashed in an unprepared organism, is a serious disorder; like cancer, it is a direct assault on personality.

If the personality tries to resist Kundalini's arousal a crisis will occur. A fully-awakened Kundalini in an unprepared individual creates no crisis; she forgets the body entirely, and the body dies. This process is much like transmitting millions of volts of electricity over a line meant to handle 110 volts. The line instantly vaporizes into its constituent atoms, no part of it remaining intact.

If, however, Kundalini is only partially awakened she will blow out your untested nervous and endocrine systems as she moves through them. If you send 220 volts over a 110-volt line, the insulation will burn through and the line may melt in a few places, but its essential integrity will remain. Unfortunately, it will not function without repair. In an unprepared human body a Kundalini surge burns the insulation off the nervous system and melts some of the body's endocrine controls. Life remains, but it is unbalanced.

In V types, or in people afflicted with Vata disturbances, Kundalini hits with the force of a hurricane or a tornado. In P types and in those with aggravated Pitta, Kundalini envelops the victim in flames. K types may resist longer, but as the crisis develops they too tumble into the fire or are buffeted by the gale. When the body is full of ama, this wind blows ama to all parts of the body, and the fire cooks the ama into virulent poison.

This is enough for most people, who instinctively realize that the danger involved in spiritual advancement is the danger of personality extinction. The fear of death of the limited identity is at the base of a Kundalini crisis. The shock of the knowledge of impending personality disintegration terrifies their unprepared personalities into retreat. Unfortunately, there is no retreat. You can't go home again once a Kundalini earthquake has demolished your home. Many sufferers from this shakti blowout exist in limbo, unable to go forward or backward, immobilized by the profundity of their fear.

The Kundalini crisis feels so uncontrollable to its victims because it is a disorder of ahamkara herself, a disorder which threatens the individual's "I-forming" capability. When your personality is undergoing dissolution, how can it properly control anything? This is why Shiva is called the god of death, and why you must make Shiva your adviser if you hope to awaken Kundalini without destroying yourself in the process.

In no other imbalance is the axiom "prevention is better than cure" more apropos. Once you are in the throes of a Kundalini crisis there is no quick remedy, no simple solution. There is no physical procedure that can reverse the energy flow and recoil the Serpent. Acupuncture can help, as can Yogic breathing techniques and Ayurvedic massage, but all these therapies are merely symptomatic. You should certainly seek professional help if Kundalini is your concern, but there is no turning back from her. You must adapt or perish.

The Ayurvedic texts state that disease first entered the world when Shiva destroyed the sacrifice of Daksha. Daksha was a great Yogi, a being so spiritually advanced that the rishis themselves officiated at his sacrifice. Shiva was forced to destroy the sacrifice because Daksha was unwilling to relinquish his attachment to his achievements. This story has a moral for everyone who works with Kundalini, because the Shiva who lives within each of us can destroy all achievements and create all diseases unless our sacrifice is unselfish.

Daksha, who believed he was powerful enough to control Kundalini with his own personality, learned to his dismay that only Shiva's personality is strong enough to provide Kundalini boundaries and direction. Because Kundalini is also the sexual energy, the story of the destruction of Daksha's sacrifice can also be read as the story of the sexual act as practiced by ordinary humans. Permitting themselves to believe that they are in complete control they enjoy sexual excitation until orgasm, when all the energy they had mobilized is suddenly projected outward. This violent cycle of manifestation and loss of energy inevitably increases Vata, and thus disease, in the organism. Control of Kundalini is possible only through control of sexual response.

Kundalini forcibly peels away puny human limitations and propels one toward a truly unlimited existence. The pineal gland is involved at this stage of personal transmutation. The pineal controls the conversion of Shukra, the male and female sex secretions, the ultimate physical expressions of the creative ahamkara, into Ojas, which forms the aura. Ahamkara must make a leap of faith for this process to succeed. She must be willing to sacrifice part of herself, part of her own existence, in order to go beyond herself and, paradoxically, to perpetuate herself. The concept of sacrifice is central to the Vedas because without sacrifice there is no transcendence, no "getting beyond yourself" into a new realm of existence.

Darkness and Light

The hormones of the pineal, melatonin in particular, help to determine how much "darkness" or "light" is present in an individual organism. They also help determine our Tastes, both in terms of food preferences and psychological moods. Seasonal affective disorder (SAD) is one form of depression that develops because of insufficient exposure to light. Light stimulation has been shown in some studies to improve such conditions as manic depression, schizophrenia, migraines and anorexia. More sunlight on your skin and in your eyes can also mean increased sex drive and fertility.

Consider one very interesting fact: you can drink more alcohol at night in a dark corner than you can during the day or in a well-lighted place. Alcohol powerfully aggrandizes ahamkara. She weakens and loses all her introspection under alcohol's influence, and proceeds to satisfy all her desires without the interference of conscience or qualm. A high melatonin level, particularly when due to insufficient exposure to light, may actually aggravate alcoholism. When the pineal is properly stimulated by light, it reduces egotism; in the darkness, the pineal stimulates selfishness. Since Ojas is produced by sacrifice, light promotes the production of Ojas; darkness, because it encourages self-indulgence, retards Ojas production.

No scientist has yet been able to isolate Ojas, for there may not be any one "ojas" in the body. Ojas may be a pattern of hormone production and release, a pattern of stimulation that inspires us to go beyond ourselves into the light of selflessness. Ojas allows the light of reality to flood the organism without obstruction. To be led "from darkness into light" is essential if one is to be led "from untruth into truth," from the untruth of selfish ahamkara-centered sensory indulgence to the truth of Ojas-producing Shukra sacrifice. Then only, when Ojas is at its zenith, can one be led "from mortality into immortality."

Tarpana

There is no permanent physical or mental cure for constitutional weaknesses. Once you have identified yourself as a V, P or K type, or as a combination of two of these, you are stuck with that constitution and all its benefits and defects until you die. Or rather, there are only two ways to escape. One escape route is open to you if you are a spiritual aspirant, and follow strict spiritual disciplines. Under such controlled conditions there will be little occasion for your constitution to display itself. It will not change, but neither will it disturb you. The other avenue to constitutional interdiction involves the ancient ritual of *Tarpana*. Related to the Sanskrit word *trpti*, which means satiation or satisfaction, Tarpana is a process of gratifying your ancestors.

There is a Law of Nature known as the *Bija Vrksha Nyaya*, the "Law of Seed and Tree." Your seeds are your genes and chromosomes, the essence of your parents' germ plasm. You are the tree, the product of those seeds. Half your genes come from one parent and half from the other. No matter how far you try to distance yourself from your parents, in space, time or interaction, your genes and their genes are identical, and they will resonate with one another. Your parents' emotions are bound to resonate with your emotions, no matter how far distant you may be from them, thanks to this fundamental identity. This explains why a certain telepathic communication can sometimes exist between parent and child.

Because your parents' genes originated in your grandparents your emotions will be influenced by their emotions, and by the emotions of your great-grandparents, and so on, back at least seven generations. Even though most of your ancestors are already dead, the subtle effects of their personalities remain in your genetic environment and continue to affect you.

Homeopathic medicine discusses *miasmas*, inherited weaknesses that are passed down from generation to generation in a family. These inherited weaknesses are referred to in Sanskrit as *Kutumba Dosha*, "faults in the family." Ayurvedic rejuvenation works on the physical manifestations of these faults. Tarpana works more deeply, reducing the emotional charges that have accumulated in you as a result of your forebears' activities.

Suppose one of your ancestors was overly fond of eating, so fond that he or she fantasized about food all day long. All cravings are forms of energy, which are broadcast into the Ether with every thought. Some of these thoughts will be rational and sensible, but many will be obsessive. You, who are permanently tuned to your ancestors' wavelengths, automatically receive these subtle broadcasts, which will induce you to become obsessive about food if you are susceptible to them.

Anyone who is really obsessive about food is likely to be thinking of food at the moment of death. This final broadcast message is more powerful than all those that went before, transmitted as it is with all the anguish of an unfillable desire. Because of the power behind this desire, and the fact that the individual organism whose rational mind could partly negate it no longer exists, this last wish affects you much more powerfully than any living wishes can.

Tarpana enables you to negate these desires. Once they are gone, the pressure on your genes to make you obsessive about food eases. Then, you can alter your diet and habits to induce other of your genes to begin to function, which can transform your emotional climate. As long as these unseen influences continue to affect you no amount of diet or routine can ever eliminate them entirely, because diet and routine do not strike at their source. 99% of human and chimpanzee genes are identical; the evident differences between our two species arise because some of these genes are expressed more than others are. You are your own creator, ceaselessly creating yourself from your own genes with the help of your physical and mental food and habits.

The traditional ritual of Tarpana is complex, but its essence is simple. It is much like the Christian All Soul's Day tradition, when people visit their relatives in the cemetery. In preparation for Tarpana consider what one food item your parent or grandparent was fondest of. Maybe it is the apple strudel your grandmother used to bake, or the ale your father used to drink. That food will act as a vehicle for your emotion.

If convenient visit the bank of a river or other body of water; if not, sit comfortably in your home, facing south. Visualize your dead ancestors, one by one, as far back as you can remember. Make each one sit in front of you. Tell them you want to help release them from any residual earthly desires they might have, then offer them a spoonful of water, a spoonful of milk, and a spoonful of sesame seeds (preferably the black variety). These offerings are the same for everyone.

Then offer a little of the special item, with the heartfelt wish that this will satisfy any residual cravings and allow that individual, wherever he or she may be, to continue progressing towards greater integration and clarity. Once you have addressed all your ancestors in turn, request them to return whence they came. Then feed the food you have offered to them to an animal, or put it into flowing water (not a drainage ditch!). It is good to repeat this process annually, preferably on the same day each year. The best days for Tarpana are New Moon Days, especially those that fall in September.

You need not even believe in reincarnation, or even life after death, to perform Tarpana. Your parents and grandparents are still alive inside you, in your genes. You are simply projecting a part of your personality, contacting it, and requesting it to be pleased with you and to relinquish any inappropriate influence it may have over you. This visualization releases you from any unhealthy psychological habits you may have as a result of the influence of these previous beings who also shared your genes, and of the images you have of those beings.

You need not even be related by blood to the people for whom you perform Tarpana. Anyone who you took as part of your family, anyone who has contributed significantly to the growth of your personality, is someone whom you can remember. Have they stopped belonging to your family simply because they are dead? No, they are still part of you, and you should remind them of the fact that they continue to be loved.

Tarpana is especially important for people you knew personally. If you really loved them you can continue to show them your love in the only physical way that remains to you: by remembering them and offering part of yourself to them as a token of your love. If your relationship with these ancestors was marred by negative emotions, Tarpana allows you to forgive them, to purify those relationships by sacrificing your negativity and offering the healing power of your love. Thankfulness for the genes which have given you life, and forgiveness for those genes which have limited your existence, transport the sacrifice to its intended target.

If you are convinced that this procedure can actually help eliminate any negativity remaining between you and the image you hold of your ancestor, it will. Faith is essential for it to work; you must make your offering with complete sincerity. Faith can truly make you whole.

Faith can also make our society whole. Tarpana is important to all of us who have forgotten our roots. It recreates the bond that should exist between us and our ancestors. Indian tradition regards Tarpana as a duty that every child must perform for its parents. When we accept this responsibility we relinquish forgetfulness. Tarpana is an act of remembrance that solidifies the link between the generations. By opening ourselves to our ancestral influences and forgiving our forebears their imperfections we open ourselves to their accumulated wisdom, which can cement our culture together again.

Conclusion

Unless you are already immortal your health is a dynamic condition, not a permanent state. There is no limit to the harmony possible in you, and no limit to the harmony you can create around yourself. Your ultimate aim should be true freedom, freedom from reliance on the external world, which can come only when you make yourself a balanced, self-sustaining cosmos. None of us who are mortal are truly free; we are all obliged to purchase our limited freedom with eternal vigilance.

We are limited by our concepts of limitation. Restructuring our personal belief systems is the key to permitting ourselves unlimited personal development. If we can learn to walk on fire without being burned, we can also learn to eliminate side-effects from therapy with powerful drugs and heal surgical wounds quickly. Ayurveda and its sister sciences provide directions for our attempts to enter into a sincere, bonded relationship with Nature, Who is the source of all faith and forgiveness. Filled with faith, we can move mountains.

Our task on this imperfect planet is to work continuously towards relative perfection. The beginning of world perfection is self-perfection. In the words of the song, "Let there be peace on earth, and let it begin with me." Self-perfection requires self-peace, which begins with elimination of your physical, mental and emotional limitations. Understanding, honesty, acceptance, forgiveness and compassion are your tools for self-development. Nature is forgiveness incarnate, and all healing comes from Nature.

Use your doshas to help you. A healthy person uses the V mode to obtain original, creative ideas, moves into the P mode to engineer the theory into a plan for actualizing it, and employs the K mode to follow through on the plan. Healthy people are well-rounded. Instead of berating yourself for your imperfections, overcome them with the help of your Inner Light.

If you are a V person, you must forgive yourself for being chaotic, for sometimes being so hyperactive that you neglect what needs to be done. If you are a P person, you must accept your innate impatience with other people and with yourself. You must never let the fact of this impatience interfere with your process of harmonizing yourself and your surroundings. If you are a K person, you must forgive yourself your complacency and be willing to move beyond it.

If you are already ill, you must be able to forgive your disease. You must forgive ahamkara for being dependent on Fat for love if you are overweight. If you have arthritis, you must forgive yourself for creating an alien servant to stiffen your joints for you. If cancer has invaded you, ahamkara must be forgiven for being so confused that she has empowered another identity to try to force her into confronting her problems. Forgiveness permits you to break free from all the things you have bitten off, chewed up and swallowed that you cannot digest. You can leave them behind you and create a new self-image. Give a new image to ahamkara to identify with, and she can create a healthy organism for you.

The prayer below can be your covenant with the universe. You offer yourself as an instrument to try to make the world a better place through whatever efforts, however meager. When you say it sincerely, Nature will offer you in return all Her powers to heal you and your environment:

> May everyone be happy
> May everyone be healthy
> May everything be holy
> May there never be disharmony of any kind, anywhere!

This is the message of Ayurveda.

Resources

For Ayurvedic books, supplements and related products:

Sushakti
1840 Iron Street, Suite C
Bellingham, WA 98225

TOLL-FREE 1 – 888 – 774 - 2584

For further information on Ayurvedic study, and
to order the Ayurvedic Home Study Course,

The Ayurvedic Institute
P.O. Box 23445
Albuquerque, NM 87192-1445
Phone 505-291-9698, fax 505-294-7572

Appendix

Khichadi - Split Mung Beans and Rice

This preparation, a common staple food for many Indians, is also a purifying, balancing diet suitable for almost everyone. It is ideal for those with poor digestion or assimilation because it is easy to digest and also assists in eliminating toxins from the system.

> *2 cups rice, preferably Indian basmati rice*
>
> *1 cup split mung beans (called "mung dal" in Indian grocery stores)*
>
> *8 to 12 cups water (depending on how liquid you want the khichadi to be)*
>
> *2 Tbsp. ghee (clarified butter)*
>
> *1 tsp. ground cumin*
>
> *1 scant tsp. ground coriander seed*
>
> *1/4 to 1/2 tsp. turmeric powder*
>
> *3 to 5 whole cardamom pods*
>
> *1 to 2 tsp. of powdered ginger*
>
> *Pinch salt or powdered kelp*
>
> *Pinch asafetida powder*

If you are unable to locate an Indian grocery store, you can substitute sprouted mung beans for the split variety. Wash off the green seed covers that split when the beans sprout. One part beans to two parts rice is the standard proportion. Those individuals with malfunctioning digestions may choose to reduce the proportion of beans to rice to 1:3, or even less. Those with stronger digestions may increase the proportion to 1:1 if they so desire.

Wash the beans and rice and soak them separately in an excess of water for at least an hour. Then discard the soak water, mix the beans and rice together, and rinse them with fresh water.

Heat gently 2 Tbsp. of ghee. While heating add the cumin, coriander, turmeric and asafetida. Sauté these spices lightly in the ghee until they are just browned but before they blacken. Add the mung beans and rice, stirring vigorously for about a minute so that some of the spices will be absorbed. Then add water, ginger, cardamom and salt or kelp, bring to a slow boil, cover, and cook until the individual grains are completely soft. Serve with yogurt for V types and extra ghee for P people. K individuals should use more spices and less water. This amount will serve five or six people.

As your digestion improves you may increase the amount of spices, and you may add onion, garlic, daikon radish or other root vegetables to the mixture before cooking begins.

Glossary

Ahamkara – literally, the "I-former." Ahamkara is that force which identifies with an individual body, mind and spirit and permits them to exist together as a living being. She is feminine because she is a portion of the creative power of Mother Nature. Uncontrolled ahamkara may, by identifying with objects that are external to the individual, create unhealthy dependencies and addictions.

Ama – a general term for internal toxins produced by improper metabolic functioning.

Amalaki – *Emblica officinalis*, the Indian gooseberry. Amalaki is the part of Triphala which best controls Pitta, and is the main ingredient in the rejuvenating jam known as Chyavana Prasha.

Anabolism – the force which causes the body to grow and develop.

Antibody – a protein that the body creates in response to a particular antigen. Antibodies, which are specific to individual antigens, help remove those antigens from the system.

Antigen – any substance which the body recognizes as foreign to it and reacts to by producing an antibody.

Aura – the subtle energy field which pervades and surrounds the human body. The human aura is produced by ojas.

Bhasma – literally, "ash." A bhasma is a metal or mineral used for therapeutic purposes after being given a number of bhavanas and incinerated.

Bhumyamalaki – *Phyllanthus niruri*, a liver-purifying herb.

Bhavana – a process for enhancing the qualities of a substance, most commonly performed with a mortar and pestle.

Bibhitaki – *Terminalia bellerica*, the ingredient in Triphala that best controls Kapha.

Brahmacharya – literally, "walking with the Creator." Brahmacharya indicates some degree of sexual restraint to promote physical, mental and spiritual health.

Bhringaraja – *Eclipta alba*, an herb which reduces Pitta and benefits the liver, the brain and the hair.

Catabolism – the force that breaks down and consumes body tissues.

Chyavana Prasha – a rejuvenating jam whose main ingredient is the Amalaki fruit.

Dhatu – literally, "that which supports the body." A dhatu is one of the seven body tissues which when well-nourished nourish ahamkara

Dosha – literally "fault" or "mistake," a dosha is one of the three forces that bind the Five Great Elements down into living flesh. The Three Doshas are Vata, Pitta and Kapha.

Emmenagogue – any substance which promotes menstrual flow.

Endometrium – the lining of the womb. The endometrium, which is replaced monthly, acts as a bed for the zygote should a woman become pregnant and is sloughed during menstruation if she does not.

Ganesha – the gentle elephant-headed deity of India who removes obstacles from the lives of his devotees.

Ghee – clarified butter, prepared by simmering unsalted butter on the lowest possible heat until all the water boils off. After straining out the milk solids the purified fat that remains is the ghee.

Guduchi – *Tinospora cordifolia*, a vine which is regarded as one of Ayurveda's best Bitter tonics.

Guggulu – *Commiphora mukul*, a gum or resin from a tree native to India and Pakistan which is used in combination with other herbs to scrape Ama from Fat, Flesh and Bone.

Haritaki – *Terminalia chebula*, the ingredient in Triphala that best controls Vata.

Katuka – *Picrorhyza kurroa*, a bitter herb that flushes bile from the liver and gall bladder.

Lakshmi – the cosmic power of physical abundance and wealth.

Laxation – the use of mild to medium-strength laxatives to encourage Pitta and Kapha to flow freely from the system.

Madhura– Sweet which must first be digested, as opposed to Madhu, Sweet which, like honey, is predigested.

Madhuvinashini – *Gymnema sylvestre*, a leaf which when chewed temporarily removes the tongue's ability to taste Sweet and reduces its ability to taste Bitter (Madhu "Sweet" + Vinashini "Destroyer").

Neem – *Azadirachta indica*, a tropical tree whose parts are very Bitter. Known in Sanskrit as *nimba*, it is used mainly in disorders of the skin and the liver.

Ojas – a hormone-like substance which is derived from Shukra. Ojas produces the aura, transmits energy from mind to body, and controls immunity.

Panchakarma – the Five Purification Methods that are used to rid the body of excess doshas. They are enema, purgation, emesis, nasal medication and bloodletting.

Parada – literally, "that which takes you beyond mortality." The metal mercury.

Pippali – *Piper longum* ("long pepper"), a cousin of black pepper used mainly for strengthening the respiratory tract, for improving the body's ability to utilize nourishment, and as an aphrodisiac.

Prajnaparadha – literally, "crime against wisdom." It signifies that perversity of mind that willfully acts in a way known to be unhealthy.

Prakriti – literally, "first action." Prakriti in Ayurveda refers to an individual's inherent "nature," the inborn tendencies that influence consciousness and activity. Prakriti determines which response your body or mind first displays to a stress.

Prana – the life force, called ki or chi in Oriental medicine.

Prasanna – literally, "satisfied, satiated." Mind, senses and soul are healthy only when they are prasanna.

Prinana – the function of Rasa Dhatu, the first of the dhatus. Prinana provides the body the kind of satisfaction that one obtains through romantic love.

Punarnava – *Boerhaavia diffusa*, an herb which purifies and rejuvenates the liver and kidneys.

Purgation – the use of medium to strong laxatives to expel excess Pitta or Kapha from the system.

Rajas – the cosmic force of activity. Excess rajas causes the mind to become overactive and unstable.

Rasa – (1) taste, especially the Six Tastes of Ayurveda. (2) the first dhatu, also called chyle or plasma, analogous to the sap of plants. (3) semen (Shukra), especially that of Lord Shiva. (4) by extension, the metal mercury. (5) emotion.

Rishi – a Seer; an immortal being able to perceive hidden realities and manifest those realities in a way comprehensible to humans. The ancient Rishis created Ayurveda out of compassion for the sufferings of humanity.

Samskara – a conditioning process. Good children are raised with the aid of cultural samskaras, and mercury is prepared for use in medicine with the help of alchemical samskaras.

Sanga Dosha – the detrimental effect on one's own consciousness experienced when one associates with selfish, unbalanced people.

Satsanga – literally, "association with the good," the act of spending one's time with someone more integrated than oneself. Satsanga actively improves one's own personality integration.

Sattva – the cosmic force of equilibrium, which is the normal balanced state of a healthy mind.

Shakti – power or energy, described as female in the ancient texts.

Shiva– the embodiment of cosmic consciousness; the god of death Who eventually rescues the individual ahamkara from self-identifying with a limited mind and body.

Shukra – a general term for all male and female reproductive fluids, and for the hormones that cause them to be secreted.

Surya Namaskara – the Sun Salute, a series of yogic exercises centering on the sun which strengthen and stabilize both mind and body.

Tamas – the cosmic force of inertia. Excess Tamas causes the mind to become dull and resistant to growth.

Tantra – derived from the root *tan*, "to weave." Tantra weaves unformed energies into form. Tantra traditionally refers to those practices that employ concentrated and refined energy for spiritual progress.

Tarpana – derived from the same root as the word *tripti*, "satiation." Tarpana is an ancient method of disentangling one's consciousness from the obstructions created by one's genetic prakriti by satiating the personality created by those genes.

Tejas – the essence of cosmic Fire, which controls the mind's digestion and is transmitted via ojas into the body's digestive system.

Triphala – "Three Fruits," a purifying and rejuvenating compound which is composed of Amalaki, Haritaki and Bibhitaki, usually in equal proportions.

Tulsi – *Ocimum sanctum* ("holy basil"), a variety of basil which is regarded as sacred and is used as medicine in fever, cancer and many other conditions.

Upanishads – a group of explanations of the purport of the Vedas delivered by rishis to their disciples.

Vedas – the ancient holy books of the Aryans; the oldest extant literary compositions of the human race.

Vipaka – the effect a substance has on an organism after it has been digested and assimilated into the system.

Virya – the "energy" of a food, medicine or poison; the enhancing or depressing effect a substance has on an individual organism's digestive power.

Vyadhikshamatva – literally, "forgiveness of disease." By extension it refers to an organism's immunity, which depends on its ability to shrug off physical and mental insults.

Yoga – from the root *yuj*, "to join." Yoga means joining or union. Traditionally, Yoga is used as a general term for the disciplines that join the individual soul to the universal soul or cosmic consciousness.

Yukti – the process of creation of a specific effect by causing a number of essential factors to come together at the right place and time. It is also derived from the root *yuj* and is described as "generated from the union of many causes."

Index

milk 19, 36, 38, 52, 54, 55, 59, 62, 63, 65-66, 70, 73, 74, 84, 109, 126, 127, 135, 137, 143, 150, 153, 177, 174, 175, 181, 189

mung beans 54, 55, 56, 59, 62, 63, 70, 119, 125

onions 21, 55, 57, 61, 162

pork 52, 54, 56, 87, 133

raw food 54-56, 126

rice 54-57, 64, 65, 66, 70, 86, 119, 120, 125, 137, 147, 170, 175

saffron 54, 65, 88, 89, 109, 165, 169, 174

salt 6, 23, 24, 53, 56, 60,62, 63, 66, 87, 88, 93, 94, 126, 141, 148, 168 ,169, 170, 171

sugar 6, 20, 27, 37, 54, 60, 62, 66, 68, 69, 69, 83, 84, 87, 114, 148, 169, 175, 178, 184

vegetables 51-54, 56, 57, 58, 60, 61, 63, 69, 88, 108, 125

wheat 54, 55, 56, 57, 60, 87, 102, 184

yogurt 53, 54, 56, 66, 74, 126, 127, 137, 143

Foods for dual prakritis 64-71

Foods for Kapha constitutions 62-64

Foods for Pitta constitutions 60-62

Foods for Vata constitutions 57-60

Foods that increase weight 87

Ganesha 184, 196

Ghee 94, 95, 103, 122, 147, 182

    in rejuvenation 165, 167, 169, 170

    See also Food items

Gold

    color 94-95

    See also Metals & Minerals

Guggulu 88-89

    for arthritis 149

Haritaki 122, 136, 169

Honey 19, 170, 172, 174, 176

    in rejuvenation 161-162, 165, 167, 169

    See also Food items

Immune system 11-12, 75, 97, 103, 113, 120, 125, 133-136, 143-145, 149-153,

Indigestion 11, 80, 115-118

Intestinal toxemia 135

Jnanamrtam Bhojanam 182

Kama 4

Kapha

    See The Three Doshas

Psyllium 87, 126-127

Rajas 13-14, 56, 116-117, 128-129, 162
Rasa 22, 24
Rasa Dhatu 74-76, 83-84, 119, 161, 171, 175
    See also Dhatu
Rasayana 165, 169, 174
    See Rejuvenation
Rejuvenation 161
    mercury-based rejuvenators 173-176
    rejuvenating formulas 167-168
    seasons 176
    virilization 162
    See also Metals & minerals
Rheumatic disease143-146
Rishis 3-5, 12-14, 35, 91, 177, 183, 184, 186

Sacrifice 53, 56, 164, 182-183, 186-187, 190
Samskaras 182
Sanskrit 182
Sattva 13, 56, 116-117, 128-129
Seers 3, 6, 7, 8
Sex 54, 80, 91-92, 127, 145, 151, 187
    in rejuvenation 162-165, 167-168
Shakti 185
Shilajit 89, 172
Shiva 166, 175, 183-187
Shukra 73-74, 79-80, 115, 161-162, 164-165, 173, 175, 187-188
The Six Tastes 19-29
    Astringent defined 20
    Bitter defined 20
    for control of doshas 25-29
    effects of 23-30
    effects of overuse 21
    effects on consciousness 24-25
    predominant emotions associated with 22-23
    Pungent defined 20
    Salty defined 20
    Sour defined 20
    Sweet defined 19
Skin 95-98, 102
Sleep 92, 109-110, 115, 117, 124, 127
Stress 113, 115-116, 125, 151, 158, 163, 176
Surya Namaskara 99, 100
Synovial fluid 144, 151